The Dizzy Cook

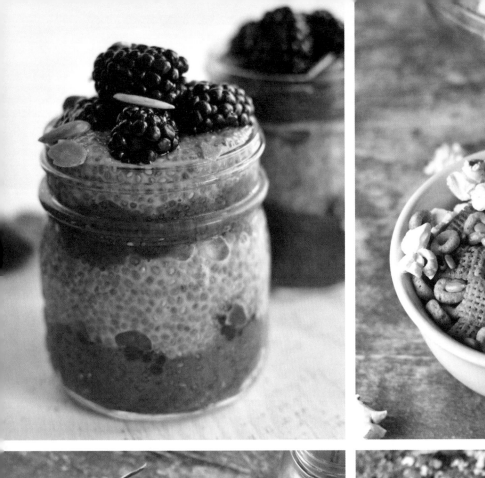
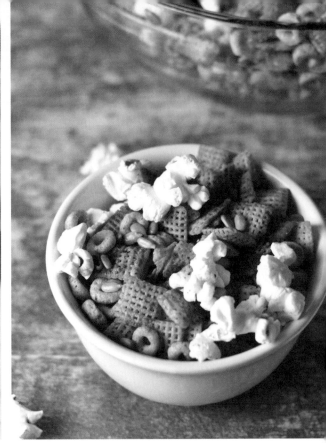
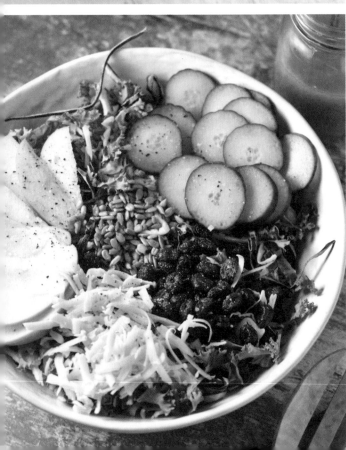
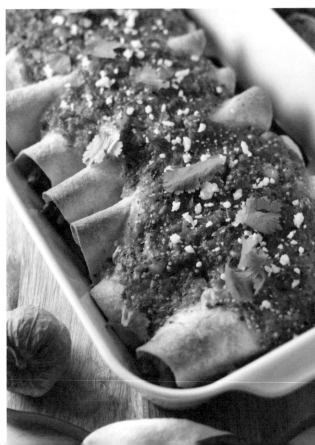

The Dizzy Cook

Managing Migraine with More Than 90 Comforting Recipes and Lifestyle Tips

ALICIA WOLF

WEST
MARGIN
PRESS

For everyone with chronic migraine and vestibular migraine disorders—
you are not alone… or crazy!

© 2020 by Alicia Wolf

Photographs by Alicia Wolf, except those by Megan Weaver on the back cover and on pages 8, 24, 73, 112, 134, 168, 200; and by Erin Tindol on page 206.

Recipes by Alicia Wolf, except those by Jennifer Bragdon on pages 50, and 208–216

Edited by Jennifer Newens and Charlotte Beal
Indexed by Elizabeth Parson

Icons from the Noun Project: gluten-free by Stefan Parnarov; vegetarian by Karolina Bt; milk by Arthur Shlain; vegan by Adrien Coquet.

Library of Congress Control Number: 2019950937

ISBN: 9781513262642 (paperback) | 9781513262659 (hardbound) | 9781513262666 (e-book)

Proudly distributed by Ingram Publisher Services

Printed in China
25 24 23 22 6 7 8 9

Published by West Margin Press

WEST
MARGIN
PRESS

WestMarginPress.com

WEST MARGIN PRESS
Publishing Director: Jennifer Newens
Marketing Manager: Angela Zbornik
Editor: Olivia Ngai
Design & Production: Rachel Lopez Metzger

Contents

LIST OF RECIPES (IN ORDER OF APPEARANCE)

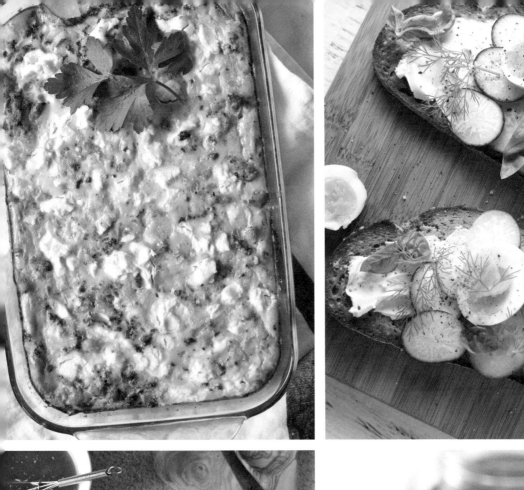
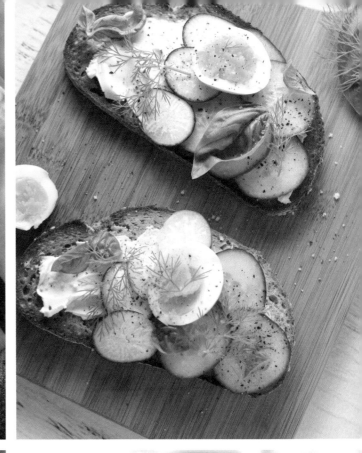
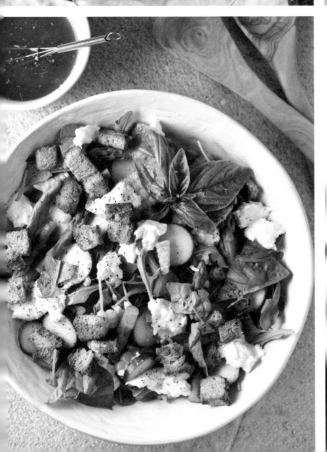
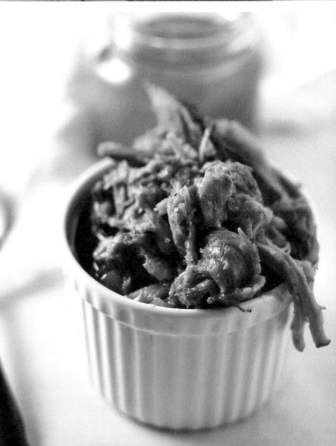

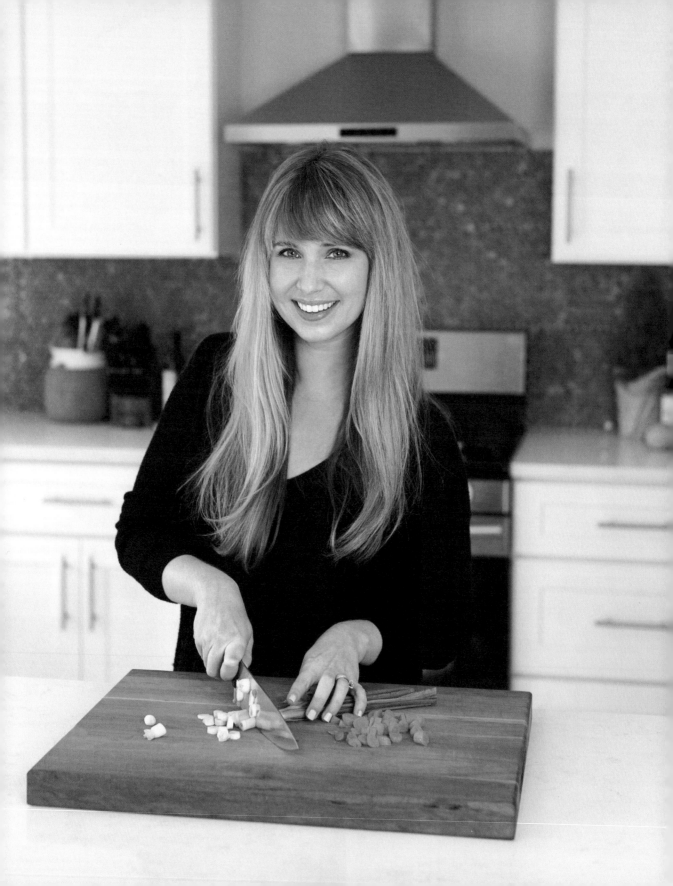

How I Became a Dizzy Cook

I can only imagine what you're thinking right now. Did I really just buy a migraine cookbook from some woman who is neither a neurologist nor a registered dietician? Yes, you did! And thank you for taking a chance on me. While I may not have a medical background, I am a chronic migraine patient and I like good food. I understand what it feels like to put every ounce of energy one has left into cooking a meal while dealing with a migraine attack. I know that the last thing you want is for that meal to be a disappointment and not leave you with a sense of accomplishment and pride for the effort you put into it. In addition, I know from experience—and loads of research—that good food can help you feel better and have fewer migraine attacks.

Let me start by telling you about my journey with migraine. A few years ago, I was a normal thirty-year-old, doing thirty-year-old things. I was working hard to get promoted at my corporate job in wristwatch development. Newly married, I had just bought my first house with my husband and we were headed off on a two-week trip to Japan, Thailand, and Hong Kong. When we returned from our trip, I dove back into work immediately. At the time, my company had trimmed down my team on the development side to just me. As a result, I was constantly overwhelmed and stressed. Between the stress and not sleeping well, I started to feel sick, but I figured it was the jet lag, and I powered through.

That next weekend we flew to a wedding in Arizona and my ears were in terrible pain during the flight. I started to feel a cold coming on and I became dizzy, but I attributed it to cold symptoms. Once my cold symptoms cleared up, I started to feel better, but the slight dizziness persisted. Over the next month, my dizziness, which I describe as a lightheaded or "floaty" feeling, progressively got worse. My primary care doctor told me it was just stress and I needed to chill out, but I knew in my heart that this was more than just stress. At one point I was driving my coworkers to lunch and I slammed on my brakes, but the car had already been put into park. I felt as if the car was moving forward when it was perfectly still.

Not wasting more time with my primary care physician, I made an appointment with a highly rated ear, nose, and throat doctor (ENT). He ran a few tests to check my hearing and make sure I didn't have Benign Paroxysmal Positional Vertigo (BPPV), a common cause of vertigo and dizziness that occurs where calcium crystals get loose in your inner ear. Because I wasn't helped by the Epley or Dix-Hallpike Maneuvers, common techniques that help BPPV sufferers, my ENT decided that I might have Vestibular Neuritis and sent me to a dizziness center for further testing. The dizziness center ran an ENG and VNG, both designed to test balance and detect weakness in the inner ear. They found a slight weakness in my left ear, indicating Vestibular Neuritis. I was given a high dose of steroids and I faithfully attended vestibular therapy four times a week. I suddenly felt a little glimmer of hope. My balance tests were improving, and I appeared to be making progress. Then it all came crashing down. My steroid taper ended, and I was even more dizzy and disorientated than when I first began treatment. At this point, I could no longer drive safely, and looking at a computer for work made me run to the bathroom.

One night, my symptoms got so bad, I was convinced I had a brain tumor. My husband and I were having dinner, and everything began to spin around me. I couldn't keep my head up. He rushed me to the ER, where they sent me for an MRI. The results all came back normal, so my diagnosis was "vertigo" and they sent me home with meclizine, an anti-nausea medication. Here's one thing I wish more doctors knew: vertigo is a symptom and not a diagnosis.

Back at the dizziness center, they suspected I had a perilymph fistula, essentially a small tear in the inner ear. They suggested an experimental surgery that would render me deaf in that ear. Again, I felt in my heart this couldn't be the answer. In my last attempt to get answers, I went back to the ENT who told me there was nothing else he could do. I also saw another neurologist who insisted I was just stressed and needed to relax—that all of this was in my head and anxiety related. Other highly recommended doctors in Dallas even turned me down as a patient after they received my lengthy paperwork.

Without a diagnosis, my employer questioned my absence. I could barely leave my bed, but it was nearly impossible to get a doctor to sign off on my Family Medical Leave Act (FMLA) approvals without a clear diagnosis. Desperate, I pleaded on social media for my friends to help me with any suggestion they had. No one I had known had ever experienced symptoms like extreme dizziness, ataxia (physical impairment), memory loss, brain fog, vertigo, and rocking/falling/swaying sensations when sitting still.

A close friend recommended Dr. Peter Weisskopf at the Mayo Clinic in Phoenix. We made the sixteen-hour drive instead of flying because of my potential "perilymph fistula" diagnosis. I spent a day in testing—hearing tests, balance tests, any kind of test you could think of! The equipment they had at the Mayo was the best I had seen in my five-month quest to figure out what was wrong with me. For the first time, I felt hopeful they would figure it out. The next morning, Dr. Weisskopf walked in. He looked at me directly and said, "You have vestibular migraine." I came back with: "That can't be possible." I rarely had headaches, and never once had pain so bad I thought it would be classified as a migraine attack. He explained that not all migraine disorders have head pain, and that they can manifest themselves in different (and very odd) ways. Some come with dizziness, vertigo, and imbalance—a migraine that affects the vestibular system. You can also be in a 24/7 continuous cycle of a migraine, which was what I was experiencing.

In a serendipitous moment, the next day I got a call from the University of Texas Southwestern Medical Center that an appointment had opened

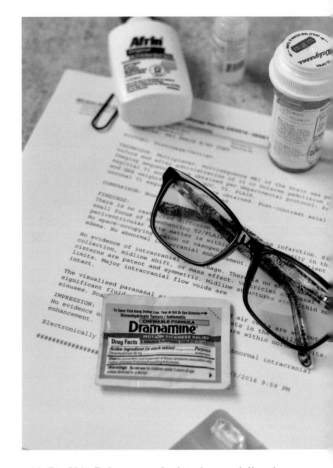

with Dr. Shin Beh, a neurologist who specializes in vestibular disorders. Word on the street was that he could solve any patient's unexplained dizziness. I had been trying to get into Dr. Beh for months, as other doctors around Dallas had told me he was one of the best doctors in the nation for the symptoms I was experiencing. But he had been booked out for about six months, and I knew I would surely lose my job by the time I could get in to see him. Luckily a friend's mom happened to work with him and let him know my story. I was curious to see if Dr. Beh would agree with the Mayo Clinic's diagnosis.

I'm sure he thought I was nuts since I brought both my mother, who is a nurse, and my husband into the room with me. This was something I started doing a few months prior when I wasn't getting answers from doctors. (Sadly, I found that many doctors took my case more seriously with my spouse in the room.) In fact, some of the physicians I saw prior to Dr. Beh would strictly talk to my husband while I was sitting right there. Having family in the examination room also allowed me to be more present at my appointment. With my brain fog, it was difficult to concentrate and ask the questions I needed to, even when they were written down.

Dr. Beh had his own set of crazy tests, a little different from the Mayo Clinic's, but he finally confirmed it was vestibular migraine. He gave me three options for medication, all with benefits and drawbacks. I chose the treatment plan that I considered to be the easiest to wean off because I wanted to start trying for a family within a few months. Dr. Beh suggested I also begin the three most researched supplements for migraine prevention: magnesium, B2, and CoQ10. While we waited for those to begin working, I began my treatment regimen.

Within just a few weeks, I was feeling slightly better, although still dizzy every day. An overachiever, I assumed I was ready to jump back into working again. I was out of paid FMLA time and knew I would never get promoted if I continued to be out of work. Sadly, being back in the bright fluorescent lights, rows of desks, and stress triggered my symptoms almost immediately. When I had to use the bathroom, I ran my fingers along the cubicles to steady myself and feel supported. Walking down long hallways always felt like I was walking on clouds or in a bouncy house. My husband was driving me to and from work most days, but on the days he couldn't, I just prayed in my car that I could get home safely.

While I was out on FMLA, my employer decided to change nearly everything about my job. They also moved my desk to a busy main walkway, where I had to face glare from outdoor windows. It was my worst nightmare. I wore tinted FL-41 lenses, as Dr. Beh instructed, but coworkers would laugh at me and ask why I was wearing sunglasses inside. I could only laugh too because it hurt so much.

To help with the stress, which always intensified my symptoms, I began to see a counselor. We worked on setting daily, weekly, and monthly goals. It took all my effort not to make these into career goals, but rather health-related goals. It could be anything like take a walk, practice mindfulness for ten minutes, or work on my vestibular therapy exercises. She had me write comments about each day in a journal so that I could review them at the end of the week or month. Looking back at some of my journal entries, it was so obvious what I needed to do, even though I didn't see it at the time. On the days I was at the office, I felt horrible. My neurologist and my counselor both urged me to try to keep my stress levels low. They suggested I do a part-time FMLA, where I take time off as needed. This seemed like a good solution to my problem since I was never quite sure when a disabling vertigo attack might happen.

The intermittent FMLA was not as easy as it seemed. I had to make a call to my insurance company any time I left my desk. There was one point where I got mixed up on my hours or days (hello, constant brain fog!) and the insurance company called me to say they couldn't approve my time. It felt as though I was constantly fighting with my HR department and my insurance company. After a long and honest conversation with myself, I decided I could not heal under this kind of stress.

There are many ways to protect yourself and work with your company to deal with migraine attacks. I just wasn't aware of them until after I had left. At that point, I'm not sure I would have even tried. I was truly exhausted. And so, I handed in my two weeks' notice. Want to know what happened after I left? They hired someone at the level I wanted to be promoted to, and then provided her with help. It was proof they wanted me out. My disability was a burden to them.

Finally, Some Hope

Losing my career to a chronic illness is one of the most devastating experiences I have faced. Old coworkers told me, "You're so lucky," in reference to me quitting, not even understanding what I was going through. I felt worthless. I lay on the couch, barely ate anything, and watched TV when I could. This state of depression can easily become a cycle if you let it. You can sit there and feel sorry for yourself, cry, and hate everyone. Or you can make a conscious decision that you will do anything and everything in your power to change it.

I decided I was too young to give up. So, I began to research everything I could on types of migraine, vestibular migraine, supplements, medications, mindfulness, and how that could all benefit me in some way. Eventually this led me to discover a book called *Heal Your Headache: The 1-2-3 Program for Taking Charge of Your Pain*, by Dr. David Buchholz.

I nearly didn't order it because of the title. After all, I didn't have "headaches." But I was happy I took a chance, and I highly recommend you read the book to gain a better understanding of the mechanism and spectrum of migraine. There's not a lot of information out there on vestibular migraine specifically, and this was the first time I even saw it mentioned in a book about migraine. Although the symptoms of vestibular migraine are different from what most people associate with migraine, the treatment plan is quite similar. In fact, there are many ways migraine can manifest itself in the body—from stomach pain to sinus symptoms. It's a sneaky illness that often makes it difficult to diagnose. And many doctors only receive four hours of education on migraine in school, hardly making them experts. Yet this illness plagues millions of people, especially women.

The book is divided into three parts: "Avoiding the 'Quick Fix,'" "Reducing Your Triggers," and "Raising Your Threshold." The idea is to reduce the dependency on triptan drugs or "quick fixes" like Excedrin, which can actually lead to more pain or dizziness days through what is called a "rebound cycle." If you're stuck in a rebound cycle,

no preventative measures will work. You must effectively break that rebound cycle to have any chance at success with alternate treatments. (*Heal Your Headache* is a little out of date when it comes to rebound information. Recent research presented from the Migraine World Summit says that even over-the-counter meds like simple analgesics—NSAIDs, acetaminophen, ibuprofen—taken more than fifteen days a month for more than three months can cause rebound. For triptans, the risk of rebound occurs when used ten days a month. Even caffeine at more than 200 milligrams a day can increase rebound symptoms.) For those with vestibular migraine, triptans aren't incredibly effective, so this may not be an issue you have to worry about.

The second part of the book covers triggers. Migraine triggers can literally be anything and are highly individual. Some find that weather, stress, and dehydration spike their symptoms, whereas others have major sensitivities to food, scents, or hormonal changes. The idea is to reduce the triggers that you do have control over, so you can better handle the ones you don't have control over. The most avoidable migraine triggers are dehydration, food, stress (to some extent), exercise, and rebound. No, this does not give you an excuse to stop exercising! You just might need to modify your routine until you can build up your tolerance by raising your migraine threshold—the third part of the book.

The idea is to raise your overall migraine threshold through preventive measures. Medications, supplements, mindfulness, activity, and a migraine diet are all great ways to do this. In fact, they work best when combined as a multimodal approach. While you may not see the benefit of any one thing, all these efforts work together to raise the threshold that it takes to have a migraine attack. For example, perhaps you previously used to get a migraine attack after one stressful day, but with these treatments it would take three stressful days to finally reach that threshold.

There was no easy way to "fix" myself. I had to focus on diligently taking my supplements, trusting that the medications I was trying were working in ways I just couldn't see, and I had to take this migraine diet seriously, even when it seemed crazy. Trust is key in this process. You're putting so much effort into healing and blindly hoping it works out. I promised myself I would give this process a few months and re-evaluate if it was the correct path.

The diet that Dr. Buchholz recommends is a low-tyramine elimination diet, where you exclude certain ingredients that are likely to trigger migraine symptoms for a period of time in order to calm down the excited neurons in the brain. (I'll explain more about this later.) Since the diet was also recommended for migraine prevention by Johns Hopkins, I decided it was worth a try. About two or three months in though, I was fed up. I had not seen a huge decrease in my dizzy days and the diet took so much effort to get used to. I greatly missed avocados and almond milk. That evening, I decided to try a little yogurt sauce with my lamb. Previously I had eaten yogurt almost every day for breakfast but had eliminated it when I began the Heal Your Headache diet. I distinctly remember sitting at the dining table and having everything start to move around me. I was having a violent vertigo attack similar to the one I had the night I went to the ER. Was yogurt really a trigger?! I couldn't believe it. Here was something I used to eat daily, but I never noticed a spike in symptoms like I had just felt. It was enough of a push to keep me going.

After that, I stayed on the diet faithfully for another four months before my symptoms subsided enough that I felt confident to reintroduce foods. In that time, I had weaned off a short-term, low dose of Ativan, which my doctor had prescribed to help settle my brain, and only took a half milligram of Valium as a rescue medication for horrible attack days, or when traveling on long car rides and flights.

The hardest part of the diet for me was the first month. I had my list of "no" foods printed out and saved to my phone, but the sneaky names for MSG (a big trigger for migraine) were tough! I never realized how many additives are in foods that I once thought were additive free. Food producers are even putting triggers like carrageenan into organic creams and milk. The diet taught me that although something is marketed as "organic" or "healthy," you still need to check the label for potential triggers. I always tell people not to count their first month because you will mess up a few times before you really get it down.

Another difficult aspect for me was the recipes. The few out there weren't very good in my opinion. I wanted comfort foods and felt deprived eating kale and bland chicken all the time. When you're tired and sick, all you want is for someone else to tell you what to do. You don't want to spend the time reading through ingredients and matching up what you can and can't have. Grocery shopping can be a giant trigger by itself, then you sit there and read every ingredient because nearly everything has additives… trust me, I know it's a beating. The thing that kept me going was knowing that if I could get through cooking a delicious and migraine-compliant meal, I could be proud of myself for that day. It was something that I made and that my family loved. Even if nothing else during that day went right with my job or doctor's appointments, everything felt right when I sat down at the dinner table with my husband. Having my family say, "Oh! This is so good!" left me with a proud feeling that I hadn't had in so long. Cooking brought the spark back to my life that my migraine disorder had once snuffed out.

Three years later, I feel as though I'm in remission or extremely close to it. Most of my days I feel 100 percent normal, and I haven't had a bad attack in months. There are a few times that the dizzies make their appearance—often after a very long day of travel, a very intense workout, or when I have a messed-up sleep schedule. It typically only lasts a moment or two, never a full day. Unlike how it used to be where I would be stuck in bed for days with a bad attack, I can carry on with my life.

When I was first diagnosed, I never imagined that I could survive a fourteen-hour plane ride or get on a boat for a snorkel trip ever again. These are all goals I've been able to successfully accomplish with the right diet, supplements, medication, and therapy. Once you discover that perfect combination of treatments, you too can get your life back.

The Heal Your Headache (HYH) Migraine Diet

There are several different migraine diets out there, but for the prevention of migraine I find the most effective to be the Heal Your Headache (HYH) diet and the Keto diet. There are a few in-between diets, like Charleston, which goes a step further than HYH to eliminate things like seeds or higher histamine foods. And many low tyramine diets, like the Johns Hopkins Headache Center Migraine Diet and the National Headache Foundation Low Tyramine Diet (both of which have similar standards to HYH), are endorsed by many as an effective tool for patients. Some claim that a combination of gluten-, dairy-, and sugar-free works best. Others say celery juice cured all their ailments. You could spend your whole life trying to find the perfect migraine diet, but it truly comes down to what you think will be the easiest for you to stick with.

Because I am a huge cheese lover, HYH seemed to be the least dramatic change I could try. The diet is based on eliminating foods that contain high amounts of tyramine, an amino acid you often find in cured meats, aged cheese, and fermented foods, which can be common migraine triggers. HYH also includes eliminating artificial sweeteners, caffeine, sulfites, and additives like monosodium glutamate. What I did not realize was that glutamate can hide under many different names other than "MSG." I learned how to read labels and quickly spot additives over time. Even now that I've reintroduced certain foods, I still tend to follow HYH. A migraine diet at the very basic level is about eating fresh, whole foods.

I'm not going to lie to you: the HYH diet is tough in the beginning. Fair warning, you'll probably have at least one breakdown in the grocery store when you realize everything you bought before has some type of additive or hidden MSG. I ask that you put those products down nicely, instead of chucking them at the migraine-free person happily adding them to their cart beside you. You want to give yourself a true chance at healing, and you won't do that if you put in half the effort. You must have an "all-in" mindset. Try focusing on all the things you can have instead of the things you can't.

Let's get the foods you should eliminate out of the way before we look at all the glorious foods that you can eat.

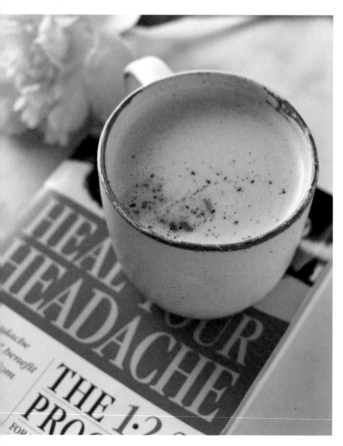

FOODS TO ELIMINATE

AGED CHEESE The more aged, the greater a trigger it could be. This includes gouda, Parmesan, cheddar, Brie, manchego, Swiss, blue… basically all the good stuff. However, there are some fresh cheeses you can still have as long as they don't have flavorings. No migraine diet is very clear on where the cut-off for length of aging should be. I find the sweet spot is around two months, which is typically how long a good-quality American cheese is aged. And the most common migraine diets generally agree that American cheese is safe for those with a migraine disorder. Fresh mozzarella (not aged or smoked), fresh goat cheese (chèvre), ricotta, cream cheese (carrageenan-free), cottage cheese (without live cultures), Boursin, and farmer's cheese all fall into the less-than-two-month category.

ALCOHOL You should abstain from alcohol at the beginning of the diet until you find some semblance of equilibrium. Once the attacks are more controlled, you can consider organic or biodynamic dry white wines, or try a filter like PureWine, which removes the sulfites and biogenic amines without adding anything to the wine. Some mass-produced wines do contain added chemicals and flavorings that appear to bring on migraine, along with sulfites and biogenic amines. White wine is typically higher in sulfites, while red wine is higher in histamine. As for spirits, vodka is best tolerated, as well as other clear distilled liquors.

ARTIFICIAL SWEETENERS Aspartame (Nutrasweet) and saccharin (Sweet'N Low) should be eliminated. Sucralose (Splenda) should be okay, but try to avoid it if you can. Naturally derived sweeteners like stevia, monk fruit, and sugar alcohols are okay in moderation.

BAKED GOODS Fresh, yeast-risen baked goods should not be consumed on this diet until after twenty-four hours have passed from baking time. Avoid all baked breads less than one day old, especially sourdough due to the fermentation. Yes, this includes yeast-risen pizza dough. You can bake or buy fresh bread and let it sit twenty-four hours, and it will be safe to eat. I prefer this, because the local baker is likely using fewer ingredients than mass-produced packaged breads. However, pre-packaged breads can be consumed immediately since they are more than twenty-four hours old. Avoid additives like "malted barley flour," as it can act like MSG. Packaged naan or pita bread is perfect for making quick pizzas but watch for yogurt in it. Yeast by itself is okay as long as you follow the twenty-four-hour rule, but yeast extract or nutritional yeast should be avoided due to glutamate. Corn or flour tortillas are safe, but be sure to read the labels and watch for any hidden types of MSG or other additives.

BEANS & PEAS Lima beans, fava beans (broad beans), navy beans, and lentils should be eliminated due to their high natural tyramine content. The same is true of fresh pea pods.

CAFFEINE This includes coffee, tea, and sodas. Unfortunately, regular decaf coffee and (most) teas should be avoided, as many contain chemical triggers and are not fully decaffeinated. The best substitute you can find are CO_2 or Swiss Water Processed decaf coffees, which are naturally processed and 99.9 percent caffeine-free. I'll go into detail about this later. Teas that are naturally caffeine-free, like green rooibos or 100 percent ginger, are good substitutes. (For more on caffeine and migraine, turn to page 229.)

Caffeine can be controversial because some people do have success with using it to abort a migraine attack, but unless you have tested this theory it should be eliminated, especially with vestibular migraine. Using large amounts of caffeine daily can even contribute to rebound headaches.

CHOCOLATE This includes organic dark and cacao nibs. Dr. Buchholz says carob is iffy, but I find that many of my readers can tolerate it quite well. White chocolate is allowed, as long as it does not contain additives. Technically, it's not really "chocolate" at all.

FERMENTED/CULTURED DAIRY PRODUCTS Yogurt (even dairy-free yogurt), kefir, and buttermilk should also be eliminated. Organic milk and cream, hemp milk, rice milk, and oat milk are all fine, but watch for additives that are used to thicken the product. Carrageenan is a definite no (see the MSG list, page 17), but gellan gum is allowable if there is no cleaner alternative (i.e., a product without any gums). I've seen people try to substitute sour cream with crème fraîche—don't do it! Crème fraîche is part buttermilk that's fermented with cream. A label that reads "live active cultures" indicates fermentation.

Note: Dairy is not considered a migraine trigger for everyone, but it can be a source of inflammation for those who are sensitive, as with gluten. If you do not have a sensitivity or allergy to it, there's no reason to eliminate it unless you find it triggers you. But take care—dairy substitutes in stores are typically made from nuts and can contain more additives than organic dairy products. I feel it's best to limit dairy, but not eliminate it unless it triggers sensitivity. If you are dairy free, Oatly oat milk is a wonderful substitute, as well as hemp and rice milk.

FERMENTED VEGETABLES Sauerkraut, kimchi, and similar foods like store-bought pickles should be eliminated since they are fermented. Quick pickles (basically cucumbers in distilled white vinegar) are easy to make and allowed on the diet.

FRUITS & JUICES Certain fruits and juices should be avoided on this diet, but there are plenty that are allowed (see page 18). Citrus fruit such as lemons, limes, grapefruit, and oranges, are considered trigger foods. Bananas, raspberries, red plums, papaya, pineapple, passion fruit, figs, dates, and avocados should all be eliminated as well. Raisins and dried fruits with sulfites must be avoided. Many people tolerate dried fruit without sulfites; you can always test them and see how you do.

LEFTOVERS Avoiding leftovers is another disappointing fact about being a migraineur. This is particularly true for meat that has been in the fridge for a few days, due to tyramine, a naturally occurring food component that builds in even "safe" foods as they age. The products of the proteins being broken down are called biogenic amines, two of which are tyramine or histamine. As foods ripen or age, these biogenic amines can increase. People with excitable nervous systems, like migraineurs, can be especially sensitive to these components. I find that this is highly specific to the individual. I can usually tolerate foods that have been left in the fridge a maximum of three days, but I have also known people who cannot even tolerate Crock-Pot meals or broth that has been simmered for several hours. If you do have leftovers, it's a good idea to freeze them right away and then thaw as needed. Keeping leftovers in the fridge for two to three days max is a fairly safe timeline to follow. Tyramine builds up in protein-rich foods where air is involved. Canned items, like tuna, are not exposed to air until they're opened, so there's less worry about tyramine build-up.

MONOSODIUM GLUTAMATE (MSG) You probably think you don't eat MSG. It's not on any of the labels! What you may not know is that MSG is considered a natural flavoring. It can be labeled under alternate names such as hydrolyzed vegetable protein, autolyzed yeast, hydrolyzed yeast, carrageenan, yeast extract, soy extracts, and protein isolate. Glutamate can also be found in natural items like mushrooms, but it seems many people are more sensitive to glutamate when it's been altered through processing. For instance, popular collagen protein supplements are packed with what's known as free glutamate acid, even if it's not on the ingredient list. See the chart on page 17 for all the MSG euphemisms and take a picture so you can reference it at the grocery store.

NUTS All kinds must go, including nut butters. Even peanuts, which are really legumes, should be eliminated. Good substitutes include sunflower seeds and sunflower seed butter, tahini, and pepitas (pumpkin seeds). All seeds are allowed. Dr. Buchholz includes coconut under nuts, but coconut can technically be classified as a drupe fruit, nut, or seed. Through all my research, I noticed coconut is allowed on a more strict migraine diet, The Charleston Diet, from the Charleston Headache and Neuroscience Center. From what

FOODS ALLOWED WITH CAUTION Other potential triggers include tomatoes and mushrooms, most likely because they have higher levels of natural glutamate. You can keep them in your diet unless you begin to notice you have a sensitivity. There are a number of other triggers that are completely individual; I've heard about red apples, red grapes, and eggs which are on the "allowed" list. Because of this, if you are not feeling a difference in the symptoms after two to three months, consider eliminating some of these items as well. However, do not let someone else's triggers get in your head. I have had great success without eliminating all these extras, and most people do as well.

I use mushrooms, tomatoes, and eggs in the recipes in this book, but for those who find they are sensitive I will also give you substitutes or the option to eliminate them from the recipe. I've also seen people with seemingly random triggers such as cinnamon, spinach, strawberries, or shellfish. These could potentially indicate an intolerance to histamine, in which case you could move to a low-histamine diet. Think of the HYH diet as a launching point for you to take in whatever direction you need to discover and eliminate your own personal triggers.

I have seen, it seems many who follow the Heal Your Headache diet can tolerate coconut well. Still, it might be best to eliminate it in the beginning unless you are dairy free and very limited in options.

ONION FAMILY Onions, onion powder, and dried onions are not allowed, but garlic, green onions, shallots, and leeks are good substitutes.

PROCESSED MEATS & FISH Aged, cured, fermented, smoked, tenderized, or marinated meats and fish must be strictly avoided, as most contain nitrates or nitrites as preservatives. These include hot dogs, ham, jerky, sausage, pepperoni, most deli meats, smoked or pickled fish, bacon, and anchovies. Beef or chicken livers also contain a high amount of tyramine. Acceptable meat and fish should be as fresh and unprocessed as possible. While uncured bacon does exist, if it's packaged it's still not considered "fresh."

SOY PRODUCTS Miso, tempeh, soy protein isolate, and soy sauce are no-no's on this diet. Soy milk and flour are less risky, but it is best to avoid them in the beginning. Soybean oil and soy lecithin are safe.

VINEGAR All types of vinegar except for distilled white vinegar should be eliminated. This is due to the fermentation, as well as potential sulfites in aged vinegars like balsamic. Technically, even distilled white vinegar is fermented, but because it is the best tolerated out of all types, it is permissible for a migraine-compliant diet.

SOURCES OF MSG

Here are names of many hidden forms of MSG and manufactured free glutamate.

Strictly Avoid
- Accent
- Ajinomoto
- Autolyzed Yeast
- Bouillon and most store-bought broths and stocks
- Calcium or Sodium Caseinate
- Carrageenan (often in heavy cream and cream cheese)
- "Fermented" or "live cultures" on an ingredient label
- Gelatin and Glutamic Acid
- Hydrolyzed Corn Gluten
- Hydrolyzed Proteins (soy, plant vegetable, etc.)
- Kombu (seaweed extract)
- Malted Barley (common in flours)
- Malt Extract
- Maltodextrin
- "Natural Flavors" or "Natural Flavoring" of any kind (chicken, beef, etc.)
- Nutritional Yeast
- "Protein Fortified"
- "Seasonings" or "spices" of any kind where they are not listed individually on the label
- Soy Protein Isolate and Concentrate
- Textured Protein
- Umami or "umami" on an ingredient label
- Yeast Extract
- Yeast Food

Consume with Caution (these affect some sensitive people)
- Citric Acid
- Guar Gum
- Xanthan Gum

FOODS TO EMBRACE

Before you say to yourself, "But I'll starve!" here is a list of many of the things you can eat.

FRUIT

Açaí
Apples–some find they tolerate green/Granny Smith best
Apricots
Blackberries
Blueberries
Boysenberries
Cantaloupe
Cherries
Cranberries
Currants
Elderberries
Goji berries
Grapes–some find they tolerate green best
Honeydew
Jackfruit
Lucuma
Mangoes
Mulberries
Nectarines
Peaches
Pears
Pomegranates
Pumpkin
Strawberries
Tamarind
Tomatillos
Tomatoes (may trigger some)
Watermelons

VEGETABLES

Artichokes
Asparagus
Beets (not marinated)
Bok Choy
Broccoli/Broccolini/ Broccoli Rabe
Brussels Sprouts
Cabbage
Carrots
Cauliflower
Celery
Chard
Chicory
Chiles
Corn
Cucumbers
Endive
Eggplants
Fennel
Green Beans
Green Onions
Jicama
Kale
Leeks
Lettuce of all kinds
Mushrooms (may trigger some)
Okra
Olives (check ingredients; may trigger some)
Parsnips
Pea Shoots and Micro Greens
Peas without the pea pod (no snow peas)
Peppers
Potatoes (all kinds)
Radishes
Rhubarb
Rutabagas
Shallots
Spinach
Sprouts
Squash of all types
Sunchokes
Turnips
Watercress
Zucchini

SEEDS

Chia
Flax
Hemp
Pepitas (pumpkin seeds) and pumpkin seed butter
Poppy
Sesame/Tahini
Sunflower and sunflower seed butter

HERBS & SPICES

Amchoor/Dried Green Mango Powder
Aniseed
Basil
Bay Leaf
Caraway
Cardamom
Cayenne
Celery Seed
Chaat Masala and Garam Masala (look for any added MSG in premixed bottles; you can also make it at home)
Chervil
Chiles, dried (all types like pasilla, guajillo)
Chili powders like regular, chipotle (watch ingredients in mixes; some contain cocoa)
Chinese Five Spice
Chives
Cilantro
Cinnamon (may trigger some sensitive to histamine)
Cloves
Coriander
Cream of Tartar
Cumin
Curry, including Thai curry pastes and powders (watch ingredients in mixes)
Dill
Fennel
Fenugreek
Garlic
Ginger
Harissa
Horseradish (fresh, not mixed with additives)
Lavender
Lemongrass
Marjoram
Mint
Mustard
Oregano of all kinds
Paprika of all kinds
Parsley
Pepper - black
Peppermint
Rosemary
Saffron
Sage
Shallots, dried
Sriracha (without sulfites, citrus, or MSG)
Sumac
Tamarind
Tarragon
Thyme
Truffle
Turmeric
Za'atar

> **LEEKS** Don't be intimidated by leeks—they're sort of like giant green onions with a mild flavor that's perfect for soups and casseroles. They will become some of your best cooking companions on this diet! You'll want to cut off and discard the thick green stems at the top, just where the dark green part starts to turn light. Separate the layers and throw them in a bowl of water to wash—they can get pretty gritty in between those layers.

DAIRY

American Cheese, deli-style (Andrew & Everett or Boar's Head)
Boursin Garlic & Fine Herbs cheese
Butter and Ghee (avoid labels with "natural flavors"; Kerrygold is a HYH-friendly brand)
Cottage Cheese (avoid "live cultures"; I like Daisy brand)
Cream Cheese (carrageenan-free)
Farmer's Cheese
Fresh Goat Cheese (chèvre)
Half & Half (watch for carrageenan)
Heavy cream (carrageenan-free)
Ice Cream (no additives; Häagen Dazs or McConnell's vanilla are good)
Mascarpone
Milk (whole milk is best)
Mozzarella, fresh (not aged, flavored, or smoked)
Queso Fresco
Ricotta (no additives)

BEANS

Black Beans
Black Eyed Peas
Garbanzos/Chickpeas
Great Northern
Kidney
Pinto

GRAINS, ETC.

Arrowroot
Buckwheat
Cassava
Cornmeal/Polenta
Cornstarch
Couscous
Farro
Millet
Oats
Rice
Sorghum
Tapioca
Wheat

DRINKS

Coffee—Certified Swiss Water Process or CO2 processed decaf coffee (see page 230 for more information)
Fresh fruit juices (see Foods to Eliminate on page 15)
Green Rooibos Tea or 100% Ginger
Sparkling Water (unflavored) with fresh juices to replace soft drinks

CONDIMENTS & STAPLES

Agave Nectar
Dijon Mustard (wine- and sulfite-free; Annie's Organic is a good brand)
Distilled White Vinegar
Honey
Jam (without lemon or gelatin)
Kosher salt
Maple Syrup
Mayonnaise—it's difficult to find a brand without lemon juice or MSG. Sir Kensington's Organic has a very small amount of lemon juice.
Molasses (unsulphured)
Oils—grapeseed, canola, olive oil, sunflower oil, sesame oil
Sriracha (without sulfites, citrus, or MSG)
Sugar (brown and granulated)
Vanilla Extract
Zhoug Sauce

About Meat, Poultry & Fish

Fresh, unflavored fish, chicken, pork, turkey, duck, beef, lamb, and shellfish are all allowed when on the HYH diet, but you still must check the labels on packaging and/or talk to your butcher and fishmonger before you buy, to ensure there are no additives. If you've ever looked closely at a label, particularly for chicken, sometimes it may read, "injected with up to X% solution" or "contains natural flavorings."

An article in the *Washington Post* from 2007 called "Crying Foul in the Debate Over 'Natural' Chicken" exposed some chicken manufacturers for injecting their "all-natural" birds with a solution that added up to 15 percent of their weight. The solution was made of salt, seaweed, and chicken broth, which the US Department of Agriculture approved as being natural ingredients. Therefore, these manufacturers were able to label their chickens as "all-natural" even though they contained this injected solution. Some of these solutions included ingredients like carrageenan, which can act like MSG for those who are sensitive to glutamate.

A phrase to look for when buying poultry is "air-chilled." My local butcher finds these words to be even more important than "organic," although having both is ideal. The USDA requires chickens to be cooled to a certain temperature for food safety. Many large corporations use the same containers filled with chlorinated water to chill their chickens, promoting cross-contamination and the absorption of water into the meat. Air-chilled chickens are separated and passed via track through different chambers of cooled air. It takes longer than a water bath, causing it to be more expensive all around. But many believe it's worth the extra cost because (1) you're not getting extra water in the meat so it will brown nicely while cooking, and (2) it's better for the flavor as you are truly getting an all-natural chicken. I encourage you to look closely at what you're buying and try out "air-chilled" chicken. You'll notice a big difference in the flavor and how well it cooks, and it's less likely to be injected with MSG-filled solutions.

How to Get Started on HYH

Right now, you might be feeling a little overwhelmed, and that is totally normal. I've seen some dramatic comments about this diet in my online support groups—but I can assure you that you will not starve, and you might even find new foods to enjoy. If you're reading this book, I know you're committed to improving your health and making the effort to feel better. Let's start with a few tips that will set you up for success.

- Make sure there's no chance you are in a rebound cycle. As discussed earlier, simple analgesics (NSAIDs like Aleve and Tylenol) can cause rebound if taken more than fifteen days a month. Combination pain relievers like Fioricet or Excedrin, ergotamines and triptans, and opioids can all lead to rebound if taken more than ten times a month for three consecutive months. Butalbital-containing Fioricet is most likely to lead to rebound and typically occurs if taken more than five times per month. If you are in rebound, nothing recommended in this book will help you. You will need to work with a headache specialist or a neurologist who is familiar with rebound to break the cycle before embarking on a diet-related symptom reduction plan.
- Get your family on board. This might require some extra cooking on your part, but I promise your family will love the majority of recipes in this book and will barely notice they are missing anything. If your family knows this diet has the potential to make you feel better and enjoy more time with them, they will support you wholeheartedly.
- To see results, you need to fully commit. There are some people who swear they don't have food triggers. While that is true for a few, I find that if I do a little digging, they eventually admit they couldn't live without coffee, or only tried the diet for a month and didn't notice any change. Or they never fully eliminated everything all at once. That's not a solid effort, and you cannot expect great results if you don't go all in. For those who have given the diet a real chance for over four to

six months without any change, it is recommended to eliminate additional potential triggers like tomatoes, mushrooms, apples, and eggs. Another option is to look into an alternative diet, like the Ketogenic diet, or focus on what might not be working with the other parts of the treatment. Perhaps trying or adding another medication, changing supplement brands, trying mindfulness or adding Cognitive Behavioral Therapy to the arsenal could be beneficial.

- Do a pantry cleanout. Get rid of all the sauces and condiments that have hidden MSG or trigger ingredients. If you can donate them to a migraine-free neighbor or friend—or a food bank—that's even better.
- Plan your meals in advance. Pick three to four recipes that interest you and make a grocery list. Because of all the sensory stimulation in the store, grocery shopping used to be a horrible trigger for

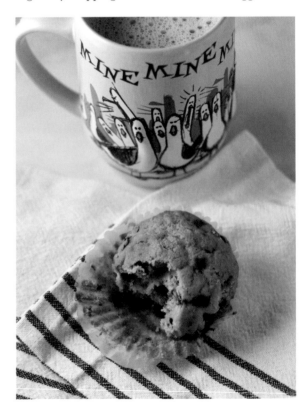

me, so I would go either first thing in the morning or later in the evening, wear a hat and FL-41 lenses (specially tinted glasses for migraine and light sensitivity), and even use earplugs or listen to music. The first trip to the store when starting this diet should be during a time when you won't feel hurried or rushed. That way, you can review all the labels and see what you are working with. There are now grocery pickup and delivery services that can make life a lot easier on bad days.

- Using your smartphone, take a picture of the Sources of MSG and Foods to Embrace lists on pages 17 and 18–19. Bring the list with you while grocery shopping so you know exactly what to look for. With time, spotting hidden MSG will get much easier and you'll be able to find the favorite migraine-friendly options quickly.

- Remember: Radical blood sugar fluctuations can trigger a migraine attack. With a diet that allows ice cream, sugar, and carbohydrates, it can be easy to get carried away and replace healthy staples with something easy to eat like chips or cookies. Eating regular meals can help control this as well as having healthy snacks readily available. If you're going to have something sweet, it can help to also make sure you're consuming something with protein along with it. For example, fruit smoothies can cause a spike in blood sugar. To balance this, you can add extra fat and fiber like sunflower seed butter and chia seeds. Hemp seeds are a good addition for protein as well. Balancing carbohydrates with protein and fat will be a recipe for success.

- Always have migraine-compliant snacks and quick meals on hand. Some good things to keep stocked in the pantry and fridge are apples and pears, sunflower seed butter, chopped vegetables, pasta, crackers, and fresh cheese.

- Know that you will mess up. And that's okay, especially in the first month, because this diet is tough to get accurate 100 percent of the time. I always say the first month doesn't really count because you're still learning how to shop and changing your habits. Just make sure if you fall off track, you immediately right yourself and try again. One bad day won't ruin the progress, but a collection of them will.

- Don't be discouraged if you don't feel better immediately. I think this is the most important thing to remember. It's easy to be frustrated when you're working so hard at something and not seeing results. The body takes time to change, especially with natural treatments. *Heal Your Headache* says to give the diet two months to start to work, then another two months to see results, but I have many friends who didn't notice results for six to nine months. Let go of that set timeline you have in your head. The goal should be to have a reduction in migraine days that you are comfortable with and maintain for a while before you reintroduce foods. This diet isn't a forever thing, it's meant to help you find your food triggers and lower your overall migraine threshold. The more my migraine symptoms improved over time, the more foods I found I could tolerate.

- If you go on vacation, try to stick with the diet without being super intense about it. Even Dr. Buchholz admits you can get away with things that you normally wouldn't, like perhaps red wine and chocolate on a trip to France. I found this to be true. When we're away from the responsibilities of home or work, often our trigger-load is low enough to accommodate a few cheat meals. Just make sure not to get too carried away. I can't really help you if you're six mai tai's in and doing the hula down the beach.

- Know that eating out is still possible! Check restaurant menus online ahead of time and ask the server questions. Most of the time you can find grilled meat, sautéed vegetables, a burger, or a salad that you can tailor to fit HYH. With salads, ask for olive oil and pepper, or even bring a small container of homemade dressing. Plain fast food burgers like Five Guys and McDonald's can be safe in a pinch. (Shocking, I know, but they don't add anything to their beef.) Chipotle is another fairly safe option. Be careful with condiments.

REINTRODUCING FOODS

It's important to note that an elimination diet isn't forever. Let's say after three to four months or longer, you're finally in a comfortable place where you feel you have control over the migraine attacks. My personal journey had me noticing a slight difference between four to six months, but the longer I kept with it, even loosely at that point, the better I felt. Either way, you will eventually get to a point where you are able to reintroduce foods to see what might trigger you. The best way to approach this is to keep a diary or notes of what food you plan to introduce that week. It's always best to start with the foods you miss the most or that are most inconvenient to not have. For me, this was avocado and lemon juice.

It's helpful to start with a modest amount of the potential trigger food the first day and then work up to more. For instance, on the first day maybe you start with a slice of avocado. If you feel great, then add a little bit more the next day—perhaps a generous topping on a salad. Then if you still feel great, try a little bit of semi-safe guacamole (avocado, cilantro, and a splash of white vinegar to keep triggers separated).

Occasionally, food triggers can present themselves up to two days later, but with such a long time it's easily confused with other factors like barometric changes, stress, or hormones. The most commonly reported period to react to a food trigger is within a few hours. What typically happens when a migraine takes a couple of days to trigger is that a person is testing multiple days in a row and, combined with other factors, the trigger load keeps stacking on itself until it overflows. This was the case for me when I tried avocado in the beginning. I found my immediate triggers were yogurt and walnuts, but avocado was so unclear. Sometimes I would get a spike in dizziness and other times I was totally fine. I decided to eliminate avocado for a while longer since it seemed to be a low trigger for me, bothering me more on days when my other triggers (weather, stress, etc.) were high. After a few months and even more improvement with my vestibular migraine, I was eventually able to reintroduce avocado successfully.

Three years later, I'm able to eat most foods that are on the "not allowed" list. Yogurt, caffeine, and most nuts continue to be triggers that I test every so often to confirm. Even though I don't always follow a migraine diet 24/7 now, I am still mindful on days when I'm stressed, traveling, or driving a long way, and my trigger threshold is low. In these cases, it helps me to be a little stricter than I otherwise would be. Even just cooking my own foods versus eating out or picking up fast food can go a long way.

REINTRODUCTION TIPS

- Start with the foods you miss the most.
- Try one new food a week, testing the ingredient for three to five days in a row.
- If you feel symptoms, consider the possibility that it might be due to other factors such as weather, hormonal changes, and stress levels, which can raise or lower the threshold for food triggers.
- If a food trigger seems unclear, take a break from the ingredient for a week and try again.
- If you think symptoms have been triggered by that ingredient, you can put it on the "no" list for now. Consider testing it again at some time in the future, because trigger sensitivity can change with time.

TIPS FOR READING LABELS

Even now that I've been able to incorporate many foods back into my diet, I still check every label before making a purchase. It's become a habit that I will be forever thankful that I learned. You see, I thought I ate healthy before, but I rarely checked ingredient lists on things like raw chicken, crackers, cream, and butter. Who would ever think there could be additives in those?

- *Check for Hidden MSG.* Take a picture of the list from this book to easily reference on the phone when you shop. MSG is present even in foods that are marketed as natural.
- *Get on the "short list."* The shorter the list of ingredients, the better. If you can't pronounce half of them, there are usually better options. Sometimes you just have to dig a little bit.
- *Sodium is important.* Although some migraine sufferers can benefit from sodium, others who struggle with a related disorder, Meniere's disease, must limit it. If you find that one serving of a food contains a hefty amount of sodium for the day (around 30 to 40 percent), it's best to skip that item. Manufacturers can sometimes try to make up for lack of freshness by adding a ton of sodium. This is why I recommend seasoning a lot of these recipes to taste.
- *Position matters.* Ingredients are listed by weight on labels, so what's at the beginning of the list will be more impactful on the symptoms than what's listed toward the end. If a trigger ingredient is near the end of the list, it most likely won't be as much of an issue. This is why mayonnaise with lemon juice as one of the last ingredients can be more tolerated than if lemon juice were at the top of the list.
- *Google is your friend.* If you can't figure out the name of an ingredient, just look it up. Often you can tell if it's linked to MSG in some way or if it's a fermented item just by doing minimal research.
- *Check the spices.* You'll want to make sure there's nothing added, even if the label doesn't state it. For example, some chili powders can add in triggers like cocoa to the mix. Same with curry powders or taco spice mixes. Be careful with ingredients that contain just "spices."
- *Organic is great, but not always necessary.* The only plus is that organic items typically have fewer additives (but not always). My standard is to choose organic for most meat, eggs, and milk products, but to let it slide on certain vegetables and fruits. Occasionally I will follow the "Dirty Dozen" List, which is put together by the Environmental Working Group (EWG), a nonprofit that ranks fruits and vegetables based on pesticide contamination. If you can buy local, that's even better. Just work with what you can afford.

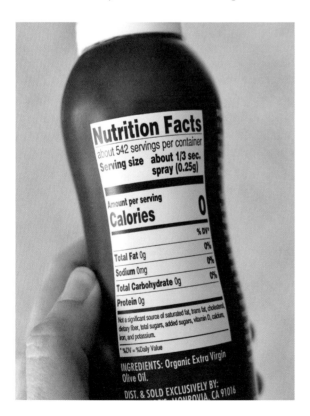

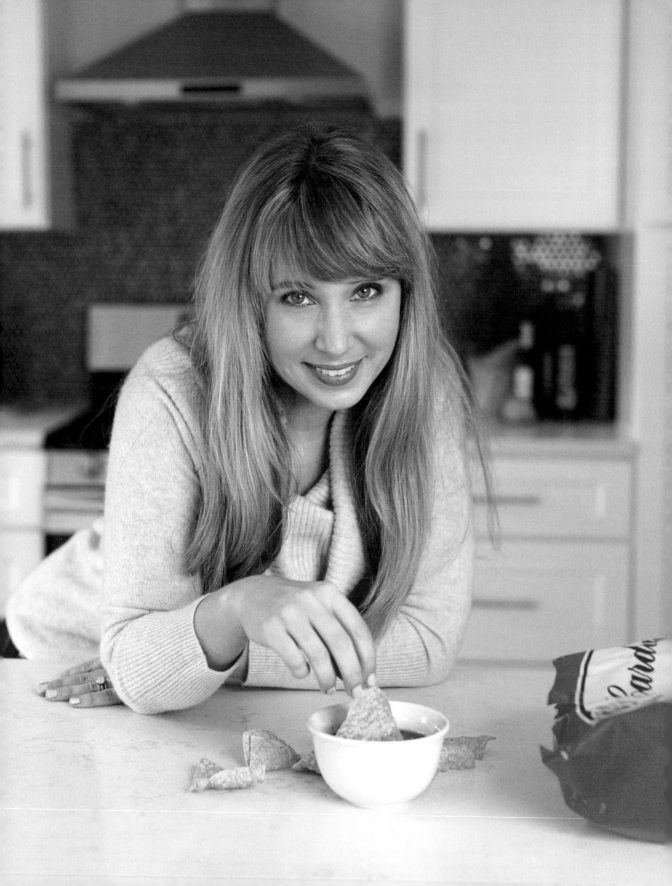

The Dizzy Cook's Approach to a Migraine Diet

Now that you've heard my story, as well as some of my tips for the diet, we are officially to the fun part. I'm not like other migraine diet cooks, I'm a cool migraine diet cook. What I mean by that is my method of recipe development is not about being the "healthiest" with zero gluten, dairy, sodium, sugar, or fun. I like to focus on how to fit a migraine diet into your life, and inevitably your family's life, as easily as possible. The goal of my recipes is to provide you with comfort and a sense of accomplishment, and to make you feel like you're not actually on a "diet." They're the kind of meals the entire family will enjoy, whether they suffer from migraine attacks or not. Trust me, if these recipes can pass the approval of my picky father who would happily eat steak and potatoes for the rest of his days, then I know they'll please even the most stubborn spouse.

I have always enjoyed cooking, but I never had someone to show me techniques while I was growing up. My mom was an excellent baker, but she was not a big fan of cooking. It wasn't until I graduated college and lived by myself that I really began to discover how much fun cooking is. Another Friday night with no date? That's cool, I'll just buy a personal-sized sirloin and learn to grill it! During this time, I fell in love with Ina Garten's Barefoot Contessa cookbooks. All the recipes were simple yet elevated. And they never failed to please everyone at the table. Granted, my friends love anything covered in butter. I also always admired Deb Perelman from Smitten Kitchen, who was a food blogger before being a food blogger was cool. Not only were Deb's recipes delicious, but she wrote about food with a lively sense of humor. That's really my approach to cooking: have fun with it and don't take it so seriously. Ironically, going on this migraine diet brought out the best in my cooking. Since I didn't have recipes to go by, I was able to push what I knew about flavors and test out ideas I normally wouldn't have.

You'll see a lot of recipes in this book that accommodate other special diets. For example, some recipes are gluten free, but others are not. I tried to eliminate gluten for a few months at the recommendation of a functional medicine doctor to see if it helped with my migraine attacks. I didn't notice a difference, but I should also note that I've been tested multiple times for gluten and dairy sensitivities that were all negative. Eliminating gluten, sugar, and dairy can decrease inflammation, so that does work for some people who are sensitive to such ingredients; however, it is not the only way you can reduce migraine attacks and I am proof of that. Still, I like to offer suggestions for those folks who are sensitive. I also have a few vegan and vegetarian friends who have tried this diet. Hopefully you'll find a few things that suit your fancy. I know the Mexican-Style Stuffed Sweet Potatoes (page 145) are a meal I could eat every single day.

I find that it's best to start slowly when it comes to elimination diets. If you're not seeing a difference after a few months, it's easier to cut things out later in the process once you get the hang of it. This way you can also make sure you're getting the proper nutrients you need. If you just cut everything out and don't know what to eat, you could be harming yourself instead of helping. For those who have additional dietary restrictions or who follow a plant-based lifestyle, please consult with a registered dietitian before starting this migraine diet. It's already restrictive and adding more layers to it can be challenging.

Lastly, if you're going to make the effort to buy groceries and get in the kitchen when you don't feel well, I've got to make sure these recipes deliver. For me, there was nothing worse than trying new migraine diet recipes and having them be terrible or flavorless. If I'm getting in that kitchen, the food I make better be good! I hope you also find that these recipes are worth the extra time and energy you put into them when you barely have anything left in the tank. When you're feeling defeated in every other way, there's nothing better than being proud of a delicious meal that you made at the end of the day.

Common Substitutions & Tips

Here are a few HYH-compliant substitutions for your favorite ingredients.

BUTTER Using good butter is important, and I favor Kerrygold since it's pure butter with no natural flavorings. Yes, you must watch for hidden MSG in butter—is nothing sacred?! Ghee (clarified butter) is another good option, particularly for those who are sensitive to milk proteins.

BUTTERMILK This is not allowed because of the fermentation, but you can make an easy substitute by combining one cup milk with one tablespoon distilled white vinegar.

CITRUS Substitutes include distilled white vinegar, lemongrass, lemon thyme, and ground sumac, to name a few. Less commonly found substitutes are tamarind, lime leaves, and lemon balm. My favorite citrus substitutes for marinades and drinks are cranberry, pomegranate, and tart cherry juices.

NUTS Seeds are the best replacement for nuts (and so underrated, in my opinion). Sunflower seeds, pepitas (pumpkin seeds), hemp seeds, sesame seeds, and chia seeds all make wonderful additions to salads. Even after I reintroduced some nuts, I find that I rarely used them. Now I almost always prefer the flavor of sunflower seeds and pepitas.

ONIONS Shallots, leeks, chives, and green onions all make smart substitutes for onions. I prefer shallots to replace red onion, and the rest I judge by flavor. Leeks and green onions have a more delicate onion flavor than shallots. I prefer leeks for soups and shallots for bolder main-course dishes. I typically use two to three small shallots to replace one onion in a recipe.

PEANUT & ALMOND BUTTER Sunflower seed butter is the ultimate replacement. I find the flavor varies greatly, so you may need to test out a few brands to see which one you prefer. My personal favorites are Trader Joe's and SunButter brand without added sugar. Tahini is another option.

SOUR CREAM OR YOGURT Try whipped cottage cheese (without live cultures). Just blend it in the food processor for a minute until smooth.

SOY SAUCE I use coconut aminos to replace soy sauce, but this product is a real gray area. Made from the sap of a coconut blossom, some brands are fermented. Most people in my groups can tolerate these well, but it's something to watch for and perhaps eliminate in the beginning if you are chronic. Coconut aminos are much sweeter than soy sauce, so you'll have to watch if a recipe calls for added sugar. I like to cut the sweetness with a little broth, salt, and toasted sesame oil.

WHITE WINE When a recipe calls for white wine, I always replace it with stock or broth. You'll find two tasty broth recipes in this book. It is nearly impossible to find a truly safe broth in stores. The closest I've come is Trader Joe's Hearty Vegetable, which has onion, but it's lower on the list of ingredients compared to others. I like to make a big batch of stock every week and freeze it. It really doesn't take as much time as you think, and you can use the leftover veggies for snacks.

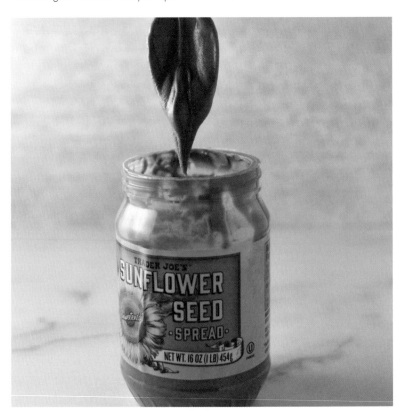

RECIPE NOTES

MY GO-TO INGREDIENTS Here are the items that I always keep on hand in my kitchen for quick migraine-compliant meals and snacks: sunflower seed butter, sunflower seeds, apples, pasta, marinara sauce (look for "sensitive" onion-free formulas), frozen vegetables and fruit, plain sparkling water, crackers and safe cheese, good butter (Kerrygold), safe Dijon mustard (wine- and sulfite-free, like Annie's Organic), Sriracha (sulfite-/additive-/citrus-free), frozen homemade stock (recipe on page 81), gluten-free oats, distilled white vinegar, and cauliflower pizza crust.

A NOTE ON FLOUR A lot of all-purpose flour contains malted barley, which acts like MSG for sensitive individuals and can therefore be a migraine trigger. Bob's Red Mill Organic Unbleached White All-Purpose is one I like to use. King Arthur's Whole Wheat Flour is another good one with just red wheat, but there are a few brands out there with simple ingredients. For gluten-free cooking, I like to keep brown rice flour, oat flour, and arrowroot powder on hand.

A NOTE ON SALT I use Diamond Crystal Kosher salt for these recipes. It's important to note that if you use the same amount of another brand of kosher salt, such as Morton, the recipes may turn out too salty. Most of these recipes you can season to taste, but in things you cannot test ahead of time (like raw meat), just cut the salt recommendation in half if you are not using the Diamond Crystal brand. Technically salt is not a migraine trigger, although some people with other vestibular disorders find it bothers them. Due to a number of vestibular migraine sufferers also having Meniere's Disease, which requires a low-sodium diet, I tend to go light on the salt. Many of these recipes will be very flavorful without added sodium.

KEY TO THE RECIPES Look for these symbols throughout the book to help you find recipes that will fit your dietary restrictions or preferences.

GLUTEN-FREE
or Gluten-Free
option

DAIRY-FREE
or Dairy-Free
option

VEGETARIAN
or Vegetarian
option

VEGAN
or Vegan option

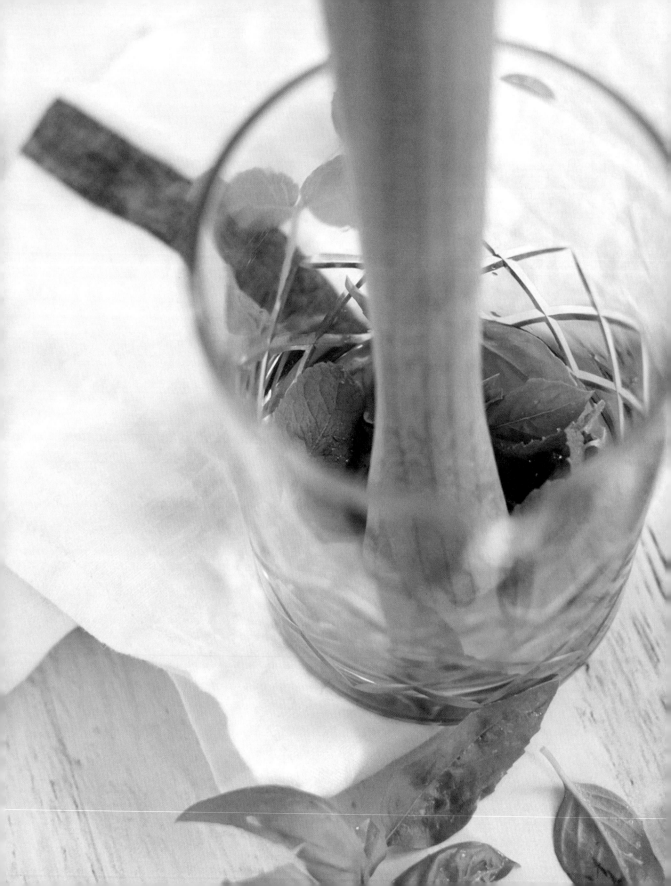

Mocktails & Drinks

Alcohol and soft drinks can be among the most difficult items for people to give up on a migraine elimination diet. Even navigating flavored waters like LaCroix can be tricky since many contain elements of citrus. To me, it's worth buying the ingredients separately so I can control exactly what I'm drinking. With these fun drinks, you can enjoy summer parties with friends or a holiday drink with your family. In fact, when I make these, I find that my friends often want what I'm having. The turmeric latte is a perfect substitute for morning coffee.

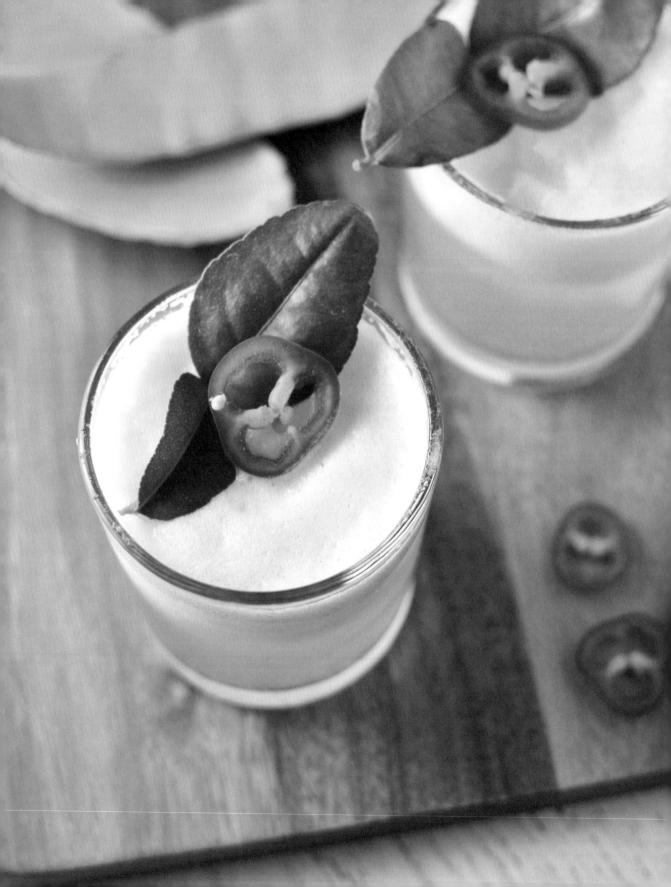

Canta-Not-Loopy "Margarita"

MAKES 2 SERVINGS

Inspired by the "Cantaloopy" cocktail at Epcot's China Pavilion, cantaloupe isn't often thought of for a cocktail. I love the fresh and refreshing flavors mixed with a hint of heat from the jalapeño. The second I tasted this, I couldn't help but think of a spicy margarita, even though it contains no tequila. Dried lime leaves can be somewhat tricky to find but are usually located with other packaged herbs in the fresh vegetable area. They are often used in Thai cooking but give a refreshing lime flavor to this drink. I love to add them in sparkling water or use the rest of the package in Thai-style curries.

---

1 cup chopped cantaloupe

Ice cubes

1 small jalapeño chile, thinly sliced (seeds and membrane discarded if you prefer less spicy)

4 dried lime leaves

Unflavored sparkling water

Put the cantaloupe in a blender and blend until smooth. Pour the cantaloupe puree through a fine-mesh strainer into a container, pressing on the puree with a rubber spatula to extract all the juice. Add ice to 2 cocktail glasses; divide the cantaloupe juice among the glasses, about 3 to 4 tablespoons per glass. Add a few jalapeño slices along with 2 lime leaves per drink. Top with sparkling water and serve.

Use any extra cantaloupe juice for a smoothie or store in the fridge for 3 to 4 days.

Pomegranate Nojito

MAKES 1 SERVING

Pretend you're on a beach vacation with this fun mocktail! Even if you can't find the lime leaves, this is still wonderful.

---

2 dried lime leaves

Small handful fresh mint leaves, plus mint sprigs for garnish

¼ cup unsweetened pomegranate juice

Ice cubes

Unflavored sparkling water

Agave nectar to taste

Edible flowers for garnish (optional)

In a cocktail glass, lightly mash the lime leaves with the mint and the pomegranate juice using a spoon or muddler. Add ice and top with sparkling water. Add agave nectar to taste. Garnish with mint sprigs and edible flowers, if desired, and serve.

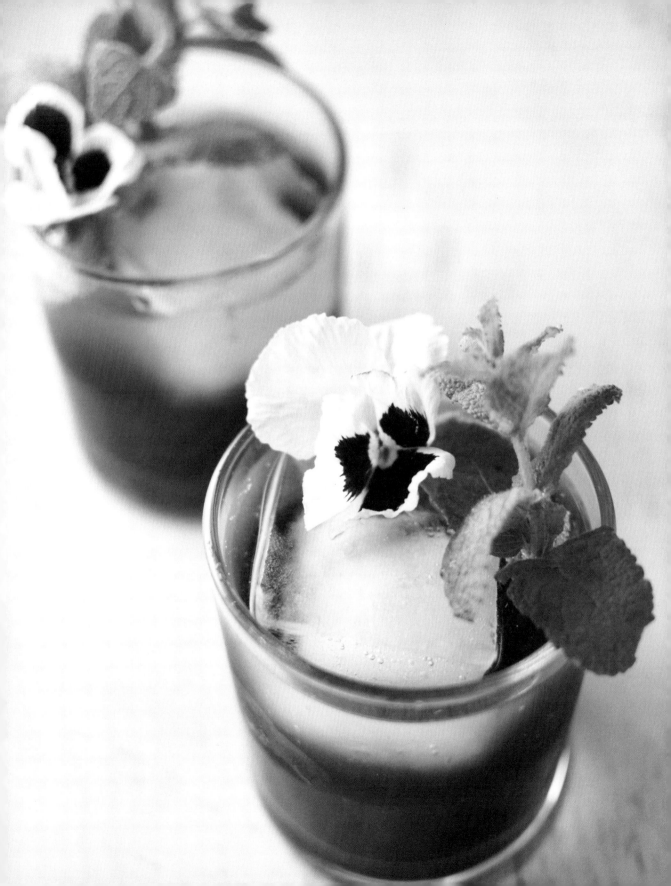

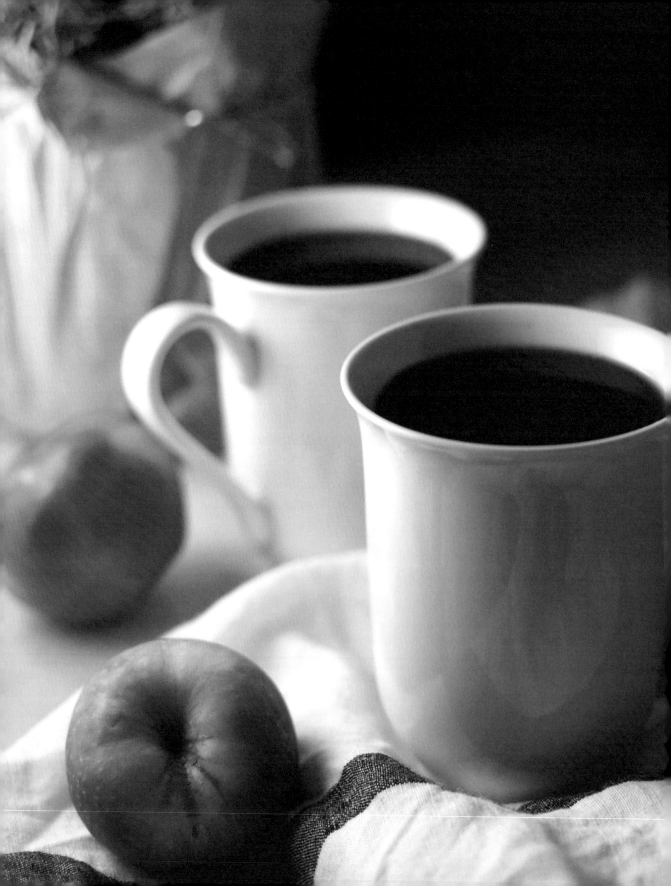

Apple-Cranberry Wassail

MAKES ABOUT 6 SERVINGS

My mom makes the traditional version of this hot drink every Christmas, but I had to give it up since it's usually filled with orange and pineapple juice. I wanted to recreate a version that was similar. As written, this recipe is really tart, which is how I remember it growing up. If you're not a big fan of tart flavors, increase the portion of apple juice and reduce the cranberry. Be sure you're buying plain juices, without sugar or flavorings added. I like to make this in my slow cooker so I can smell the spices all day, but the stovetop works fine too.

---

3 cups apple juice (preferably Honeycrisp)

1½ cups cranberry juice

3 cinnamon sticks

1 teaspoon whole cloves

1 tablespoon honey

1 Honeycrisp apple, sliced (top, bottom, and seeds discarded)

In a slow cooker or saucepan, combine the apple juice, cranberry juice, cinnamon sticks, cloves, and honey. Float the apple slices on top. Set the slow cooker on low heat for 3 hours or simmer on the stove 30 to 40 minutes. Remove the cloves, cinnamon sticks, and apples before serving unless you don't mind fishing around to avoid them. Ladle the wassail into mugs and serve hot.

Golden Spiced Latte

MAKES 1 SERVING

My favorite milk substitute for lattes is oat milk because it gets nice and frothy. Oatly is a good brand, but you can also make your own at home by blending oats with water.

---

1 cup milk or oat milk

1 teaspoon maple syrup
or honey

½ teaspoon ground turmeric,
plus more for garnish,
if desired

¼ teaspoon ground cardamom

¼ teaspoon vanilla extract

Freshly ground black pepper

In a small saucepan, warm the milk until it just barely begins to simmer. Stir in the maple syrup, turmeric, cardamom, and vanilla, then carefully transfer to a blender. Blend on high speed for 30 to 40 seconds until frothy (you can also use an electric milk frother if you have one). Pour the mixture into a mug, top with pepper and a little pinch of turmeric, if desired, and serve hot.

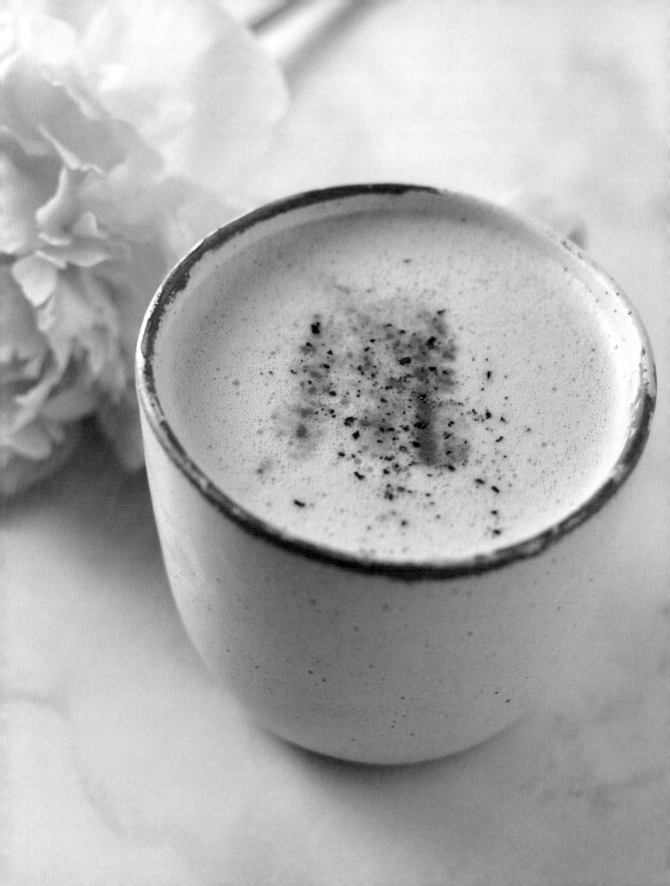

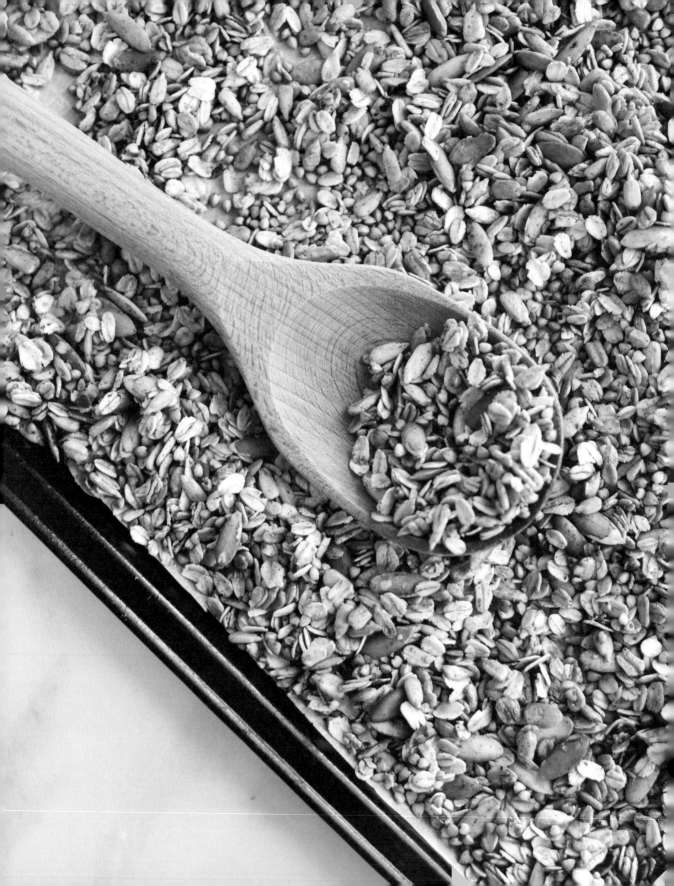

Breakfast

I find breakfast to be one of the most challenging aspects of a migraine diet. The typical American breakfast would include eggs with cheddar cheese, bacon or sausage, and a big cup of coffee. Pre-packaged bacon and sausage, even uncured and nitrate-free, can still be high in tyramine since it's not necessarily fresh. Occasionally, you can get lucky with finding safe sausage at the grocery store or local butcher. Ask your butcher to help you find compliant fresh ones, not in the packaged area.

The breakfasts in this chapter cover a multitude of needs. If I'm having a busy week or not feeling well, I'll prep the chia seed pudding or overnight oats to have ready for something quick and light. The sausage balls are another great recipe to have on hand for extra protein on the go. Keep them in your freezer and thaw as you need them. If I have a little more time, the Faux-Yo Açaí Bowl hits my cravings for yogurt and berries. When I top it with the Crunchy Buckwheat Granola, it's one of my favorite breakfasts of all time. The granola also makes a fantastic snack.

For special occasions, I love making the Leek & Goat Cheese Breakfast Casserole. It's something the whole family will love. But if you don't have the time for it, the Blueberry Muffins can easily be frozen and thawed.

Although eggs are allowed on a migraine diet, some people do better when they're baked into things versus on their own. That's why you'll find most of these recipes have baked eggs or have a vegan option. Eggs are high in riboflavin (B2), which is a natural migraine preventative, so it's good to include them in your diet if you can tolerate them. It's best to buy organic, pasture-raised eggs. I can even tell a difference in taste when my friend brings me fresh eggs from her chicken coop. Unfortunately, we don't all have access to the best eggs out there, so with many of these recipes I wanted to focus on quick and easy, with minimal triggers.

And don't rule out the Baked Bean Taquitos for a grab-and-go breakfast (or snack) that's super flavorful. Changing the way we look at breakfast and letting go of traditional meals can open up so many possibilities.

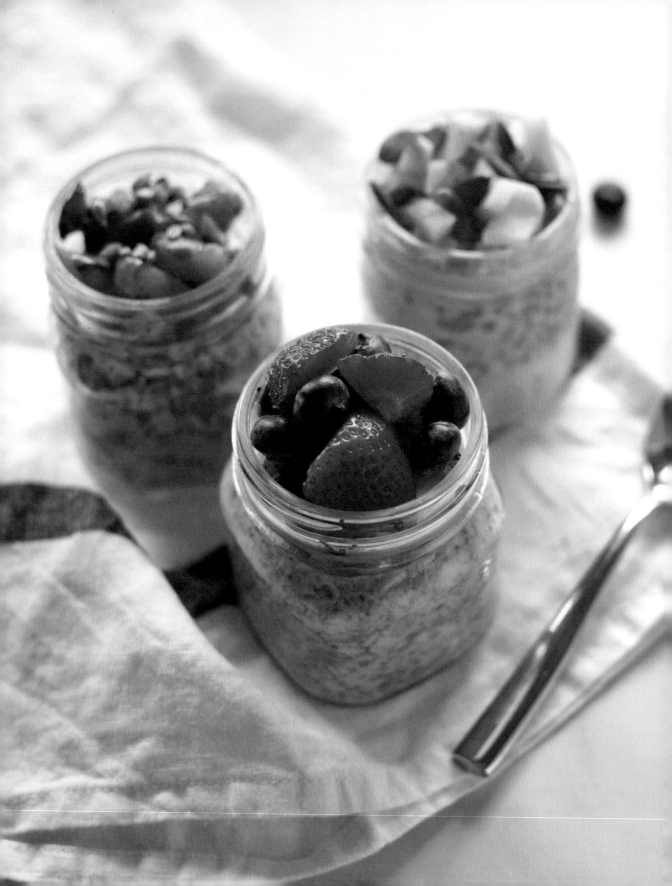

Overnight Oats Three Ways

MAKES 1 SERVING EACH

The ultimate make-ahead breakfast, overnight oats have been done a million different ways. With these recipes, I wanted to bring you something unique. The basic overnight oats with berries and sunflower seed butter are for days you don't want to think about breakfast. On other days, you have the healthy option of turmeric- and ginger-spiced oats. Finally, you have oats topped with buttery cinnamon pears for those days when you're feeling a little decadent. Using homemade hemp milk (see sidebar) is a great way to get extra protein in addition to the sunflower seed butter. Each recipe makes one serving, but they're easily multiplied to make more. Use certified gluten-free oats if desired.

½ cup rolled oats
½ cup milk of your choice

BASIC OVERNIGHT OATS
1 tablespoon sunflower seed butter
2 teaspoons chia seeds
1 teaspoon vanilla extract
1 teaspoon honey or maple syrup (optional)
Berries of your choice
Sunflower, chia, and/or pepitas (pumpkin seeds) for topping

TURMERIC-GINGER OATS
2 teaspoons chia seeds
½ teaspoon maple syrup or honey
¼ teaspoon ground ginger
¼ teaspoon ground turmeric
1 small apple

CINNAMON-PEAR OATS
2 teaspoons chia seeds
1 teaspoon vanilla extract
1 small Bartlett pear
1 tablespoon unsalted butter
½ teaspoon ground cinnamon

For any of the overnight oats, combine the oats and milk in a container.

To make the Basic Overnight Oats, add the sunflower seed butter, chia seeds, vanilla, and honey (if using) to the oat mixture and give it a good stir. Cover and refrigerate overnight or at least 4 hours. The longer the oats and chia seeds soak, the softer they will be. In the morning, stir again, add berries of choice, top with seeds, and serve.

To make the Turmeric-Ginger Overnight Oats, add the chia seeds, maple syrup, ginger, and turmeric to the oat mixture and give it a good stir. Cover and refrigerate overnight or at least 4 hours. The longer the oats and chia seeds soak, the softer they will be. In the morning, dice the apple, stir it into the oats, and serve.

To make the Cinnamon-Pear Overnight Oats, add the chia seeds and vanilla to the oat mixture and give it a good stir. Cover and refrigerate overnight or at least 4 hours. The longer the oats and chia seeds soak, the softer they will be. In the morning, dice the pear and sauté it in a small skillet with butter over medium heat. Stir in the cinnamon. Top the oats with the warm cinnamon pears and serve.

> **HOMEMADE HEMP MILK** Here's my recipe: Place ½ cup shelled raw hemp seeds, 3 cups filtered water, 1 teaspoon vanilla extract, and a sweetener like lucuma powder (to taste) in a blender. Blend on high speed for 1 minute until smooth. Chill.

Faux-Yo Açaí Bowl

MAKES 1 LARGE BOWL OR 2 SMALL PARFAITS

I love an açaí bowl, but it's tough to find ones that don't contain bananas or yogurt. I used to make mine with just berries, but they were always missing that creamy texture. That's when I had the crazy idea to try frozen riced cauliflower. I know, it's a little strange, but trust me when I say it adds a perfect velvety texture and cuts the sweetness just the right amount. A little buckwheat granola on top makes this one of my favorite migraine-safe breakfasts. Feel free to substitute frozen berries for cherries to mix up the flavor.

---

1 packet (3.5 ounces or 100 grams) frozen açaí or 2 teaspoons açaí powder

⅓ cup frozen riced cauliflower

½ cup frozen pitted red cherries

½ cup milk of choice

1 tablespoon sunflower seed butter

2 teaspoons chia seeds

1 teaspoon vanilla extract

2 teaspoons honey or maple syrup (optional)

Fresh migraine-safe fruit (strawberries, blueberries, blackberries)

Crunchy Buckwheat Granola (page 45) to taste

In a high-speed blender, combine the açaí, frozen cauliflower, frozen cherries, milk, sunflower seed butter, chia seeds, vanilla, and sweetener (if using). Blend on low speed, slowly increasing to high. Because of the thickness of the mixture, a tamper may need to be used to thoroughly combine the ingredients without making the smoothie too thin. Spoon mixture into a bowl or parfait cups, top with fresh fruit and granola, and serve immediately.

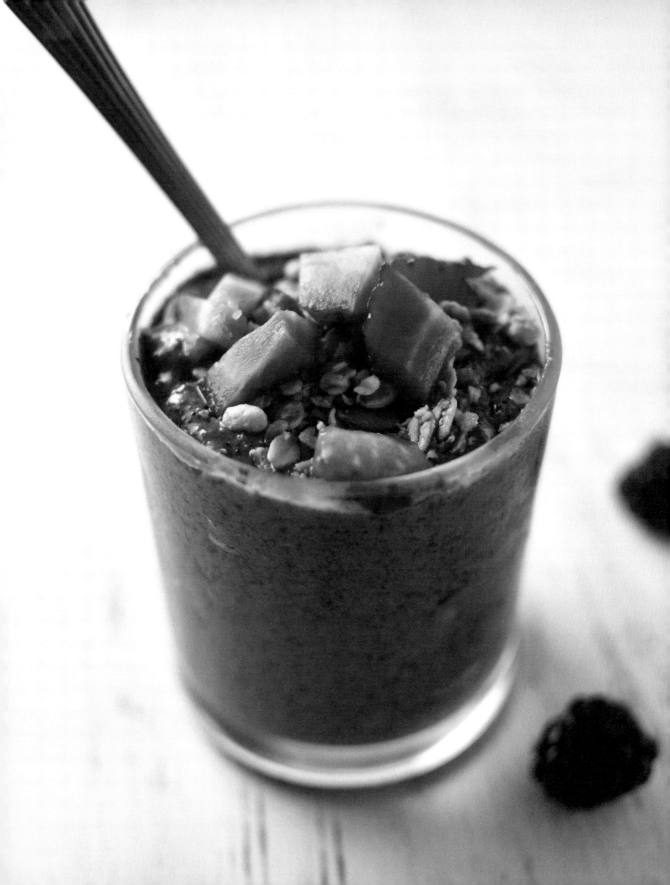

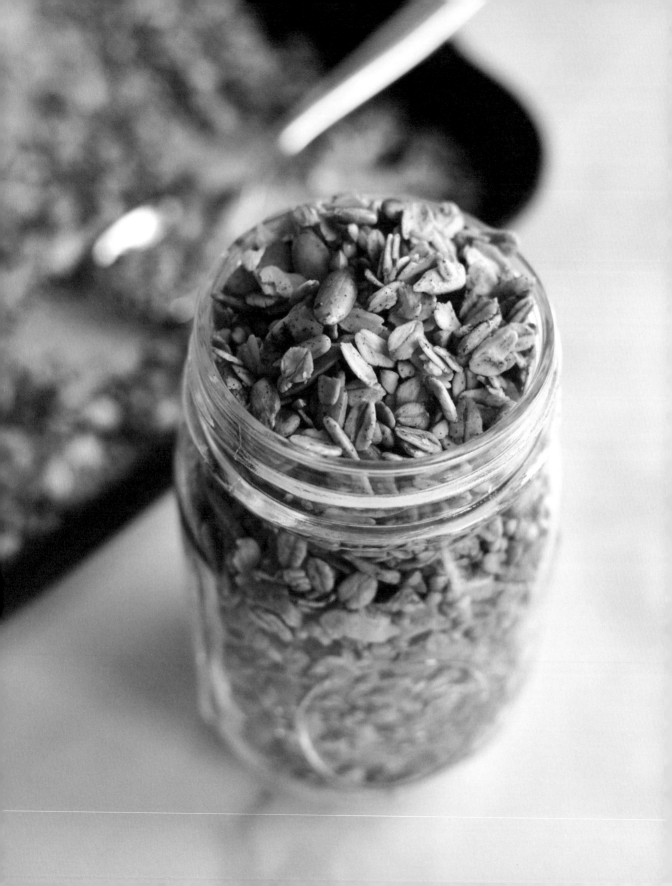

Crunchy Buckwheat Granola

MAKES ABOUT 3 CUPS

This slightly salty, not-too-sweet granola is addictive. I never really liked any of the granola recipes out there—they were all too sweet, had too many oats or nuts, or weren't crunchy enough. Clearly, I have high granola standards. I set out to create my own recipe thinking buckwheat would make an interesting option to add a little crunch. The first time I did, I grabbed toasted buckwheat, otherwise known as kasha, assuming it would be more flavorful. Let me tell you, eating kasha is like eating rocks. So, if you make this recipe, I highly recommend using plain, untoasted buckwheat groats—unless you really like seeing the dentist. For a vegan option, replace the honey with maple syrup.

1½ cups rolled oats, certified gluten-free, if desired

¾ cup raw buckwheat groats

½ cup raw pepitas (pumpkin seeds)

½ cup raw sunflower seeds

3 tablespoons unsalted butter, melted, or neutral oil

3 tablespoons honey or maple syrup

1 teaspoon ground cinnamon

1 teaspoon vanilla extract

¼ teaspoon kosher salt

Preheat the oven to 300°F.

In a large bowl, stir together the oats, buckwheat groats, pepitas, and sunflower seeds. Add the butter or oil, honey or maple syrup, cinnamon, vanilla, and salt. Stir to combine.

Line a large baking sheet with parchment paper and spread the granola mixture out in an even layer. Bake the granola until evenly toasted, about 45 minutes, stirring every 15 minutes and spreading it back out.

Remove the granola from the oven and allow it to cool. The granola can be stored in an airtight container at room temperature or in the refrigerator for up to 1 month… but it never lasts that long.

> **SUBSTITUTION TIP** Most cooking oils are so refined that even types like peanut or avocado should not be a migraine trigger. However, if you do have a sensitivity, you can always substitute another neutral oil, melted butter, or melted ghee.

Green Eggs No Ham (Shakshuka Verde)

MAKES 2 TO 4 SERVINGS

Tomatillos are one of my favorite migraine diet foods because they have a naturally tangy flavor, which helps quell the craving for vinegar or citrus. People often confuse them with green tomatoes (unripe tomatoes), but they actually come from a different plant. Tomatillos have a papery husk on the outside that you peel away to reveal a bright green fruit. An 11-ounce can of tomatillos is equal to one pound of fresh, but this recipe is best when using fresh (basically the ultimate rule of a migraine diet). Shakshuka is a breakfast food in Israel that first originated in North Africa and is traditionally made with red pepper and tomatoes. Although the classic version is always amazing, I love putting a Texan twist on it. You'll need some tortilla chips or pita bread for scooping up the tasty sauce.

---

1 pound fresh tomatillos, outer husks removed

3 cloves garlic, unpeeled

1 small shallot, peeled and quartered

½ jalapeño, seeded and stem removed

⅓ cup chopped fresh cilantro

½ teaspoon ground cumin

½ teaspoon kosher salt

4–5 large eggs

Tortilla chips or pita bread (made without yogurt) for serving

Fresh parsley or cilantro leaves for garnish (optional)

Heat the broiler and position the oven rack about 6 inches from the heat source. Put the second oven rack in the center of the oven. Wash the tomatillos under warm water to remove the sticky residue and pat them dry. Remove the top stem from each tomatillo and place them stem side down on a baking sheet along with the unpeeled garlic cloves, shallot, and jalapeño. Broil on the upper rack for 7 to 10 minutes, checking to make sure the garlic and jalapeño don't burn. You should have a few black splotches on everything.

Remove the vegetables from the oven and heat the oven to 375°F. Peel the garlic, which should be soft. Add to a blender or food processor along with the broiled tomatillos, shallots, and jalapeño. Add cilantro, cumin, and salt. Blend until smooth.

Pour the blended tomatillo sauce into a large cast-iron skillet (or other oven-safe skillet). With a spoon, make 4 to 5 small divots in the sauce for the eggs. Crack the eggs one at a time, gently setting them into the divots. Put the pan in the oven on the middle rack and bake until the egg whites are opaque, the yolks are still slightly runny, and the sauce is bubbling, about 10 minutes. If desired, garnish with fresh herb leaves. Serve warm with pita bread or tortilla chips.

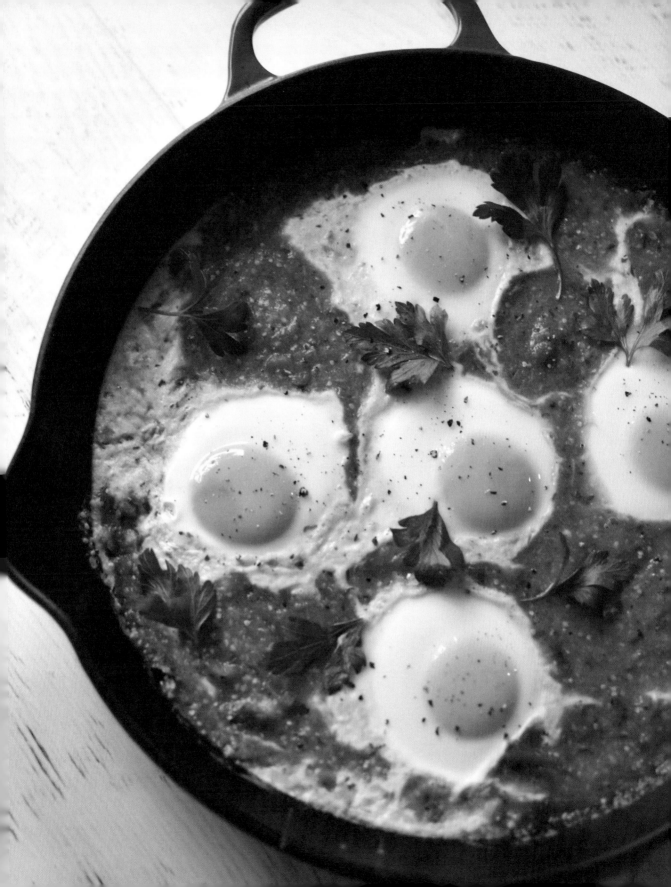

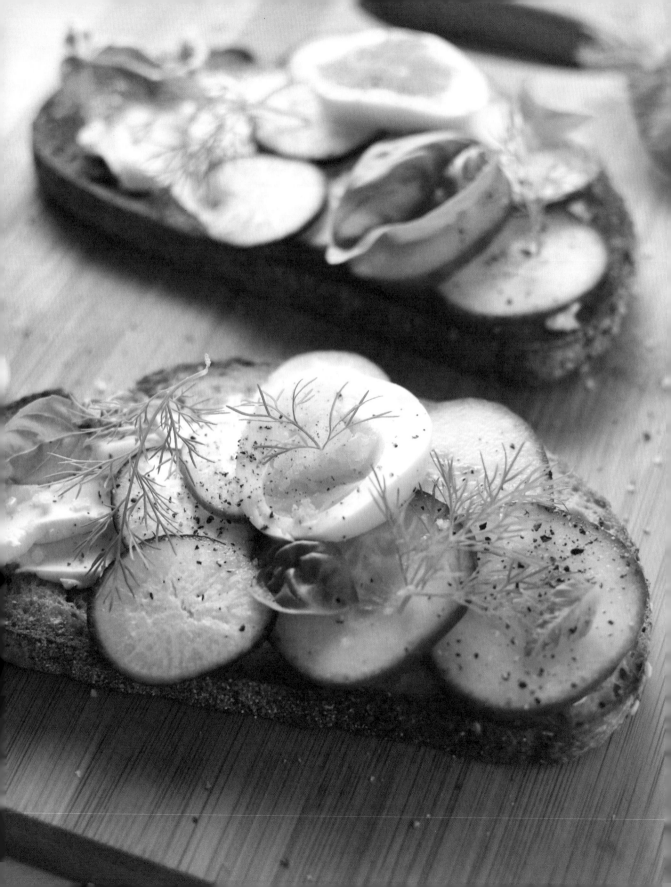

Better-Than-Avocado Toast

MAKES 1 SERVING

I hate eating the same thing every day—it's why I can't stand leftovers. But when I travel, I don't have a ton of options when it comes to HYH-compliant meals. This recipe was born from that predicament. I was visiting family and tired of oatmeal with berries, but there weren't a ton of other choices that would fit my diet. Grabbing every migraine-safe item I could, I lined up bread, cream cheese, fresh herbs, an egg, and some cucumber. After my first bite, I couldn't believe I had lived for thirty years without trying this combination. If you are missing avocado toast, give this one a try. You might not miss it anymore.

---

1 large egg

1–2 slices of bread (gluten-free, if desired), toasted

1–2 tablespoons cream cheese (carrageenan-free)

Sliced cucumber

Sliced radish

Handful of chopped fresh herbs (dill, basil, and parsley are some of my favorites)

Kosher salt and freshly ground black pepper

Bring a small pot of water to boil over high heat, then reduce the heat to low. Gently place the egg in the water, then cover the pot and increase the heat to medium so that the water just boils. Boil for 12 to 14 minutes for a hardboiled egg, or 6 to 7 minutes for a softer yolk. While you wait, prepare a bowl of ice water. Once the time is up, immediately put the egg into the ice water, wait a minute or two, then peel and slice or chop the egg.

Spread the toasted bread with cream cheese, then top with cucumber, radish, herbs, and the egg. Sprinkle with salt and pepper. Serve immediately.

MIGRAINE-SAFE BREAD To find migraine-safe bread in stores, look for varieties without malted barley and those that have few ingredients on the label. Dave's Killer Bread, some versions of Manna Bread, and Pepperidge Farm Wheat are good options that are well tolerated. For gluten-free eaters, finding head-friendly bread is tough. Free Bread is good but contains xanthan gum, and Against the Grain Original Rolls are compliant, but your best bet is to look for a loaf from a local bakery. Be sure to check if they are using nut flours. Also, if xanthan gum triggers you, gluten-free bread may be out of reach. Some cream cheese can contain quite a few triggers like carrageenan. Organic Valley and Arla are good options.

The Dizzy Baker's Famous Blueberry Muffins

MAKES 12 MUFFINS

I met Jennifer Bragdon through one of my favorite support groups, Migraine Strong. Like me, she was diagnosed with vestibular migraine and her journey was similar to mine. We began to chat over Messenger and became good friends. Having someone who knows exactly what you're going through is invaluable, and I'll always be thankful for her. I noticed she would post this recipe in the group as a yummy breakfast option, and people always raved that they were the best muffins ever. When I started The Dizzy Cook, I asked Jennifer to guest post these famous muffins. People loved them so much, she eventually became a regular as the "The Dizzy Baker," with a monthly post of fresh goodies. I just couldn't do a cookbook without featuring these guys… and her! Jennifer says that this recipe would work wonderfully with other migraine-safe fruit that's in season, like blackberries. Find out more about Jennifer, her story, and her delicious recipes on pages 206–217.

---

1 cup certified gluten-free oat flour

1 cup brown rice flour

½ cup white cane sugar, plus more for sprinkling

2 teaspoons baking powder

½ teaspoon kosher salt

½ cup unsalted butter, at room temperature

½ cup milk

2 large eggs

1 teaspoon vanilla extract

2 cups fresh or frozen blueberries

Preheat the oven to 375°F. Line a 12-cup muffin pan with paper liners.

Combine the oat flour, brown rice flour, sugar, baking powder, and salt in a large bowl. Add the butter, milk, eggs, and vanilla. Stir with a rubber spatula to combine, but do not overmix. Fold the blueberries into the batter until just incorporated. Divide evenly among muffin cups. Sprinkle a little extra sugar on top of each muffin for some added crunch.

Bake until a toothpick inserted in the center comes out clean, about 40 minutes. Let cool on a wire rack before serving.

Note: If you want to substitute regular flour for the gluten-free flour, decrease the baking time to 30 to 35 minutes.

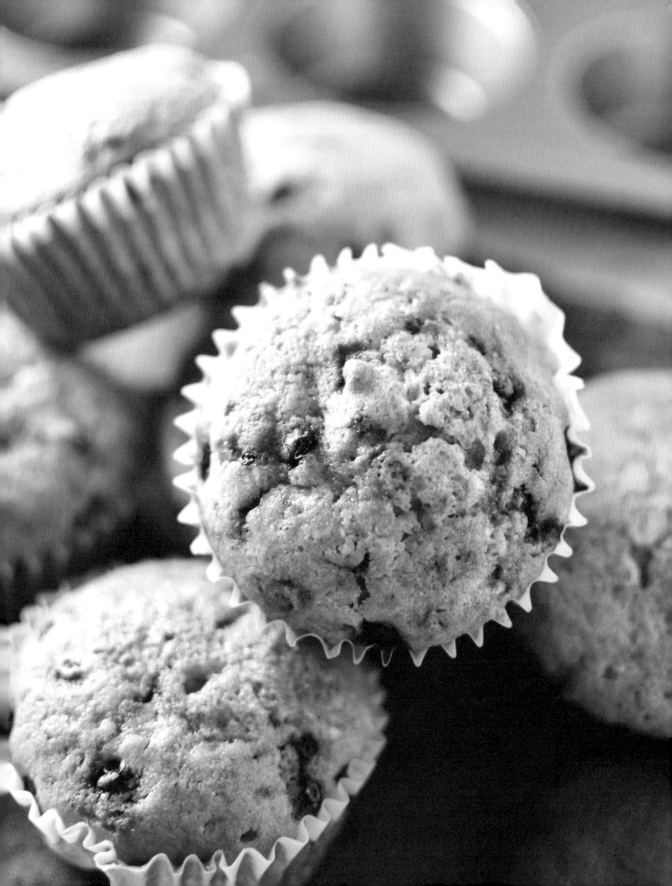

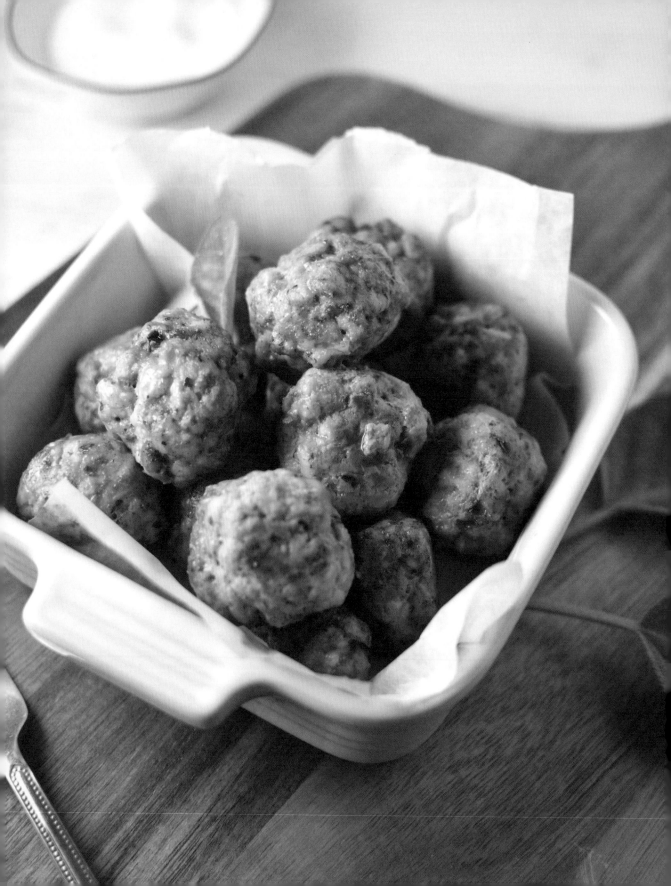

Sausage Balls

MAKES ABOUT SIXTEEN 1½-INCH BALLS

Most store-bought sausage contains MSG and other preservatives or is high in tyramine since it was probably made in advance. Some of us are lucky enough to have good butchers that offer fresh, migraine-friendly options, but I wanted to create an easy breakfast sausage recipe that anyone could whip up easily. I got the idea for these from a recipe I used to make for Christmas parties: Southern Sausage Balls. They were not healthy or migraine safe, but always super-delicious and a hit at any party. At the very basic level, I realized anything in ball form is fun to eat. They're simple to cook, they freeze beautifully, and they make a great building block for main dishes.

---

1 pound freshly ground pork or chicken thigh meat

1 teaspoon garlic powder

1 teaspoon dried marjoram

1 teaspoon ground sage

½ teaspoon kosher salt

⅛–¼ teaspoon crushed red pepper flakes (use more if you like a little heat)

In a bowl, combine the pork, garlic powder, marjoram, sage, salt, and red pepper. Using clean hands, mix until the ingredients are uniformly dispersed. Cover and refrigerate for at least 30 minutes and up to 24 hours. The longer you allow the meat to sit with the spices, the more flavorful it will become.

Preheat the oven to 400°F. Line a baking sheet with parchment paper. Form the meat mixture into roughly 1½-inch balls and place on the sheet 1 inch apart. Bake until browned and cooked through, 18 to 20 minutes. Serve warm.

You can freeze these and reheat them by covering them in foil and baking at 300°F for 15 minutes.

Leek & Goat Cheese Breakfast Casserole

MAKES 8 SERVINGS

I'll admit, I've never been a huge breakfast casserole person. Oftentimes, they feel heavy and that's not the way I like to start my mornings. But when the parents come for Christmas, I cannot be caught serving açai bowls, or my dad will exclaim, "Bah humbug!" I tested out this recipe for Christmas last year and was surprised by how much I loved it. Goat cheese gives this a wonderful flavor that seems so elegant compared to a not-so-head-safe cheddar. And using fresh chicken sausage makes this meal a little bit lighter than using traditional pork sausage.

1–2 Yukon Gold potatoes, skin on, scrubbed, and cut into ½-inch cubes (about 1½ cups)

1 tablespoon extra-virgin olive oil, plus more for greasing pan

½ pound (half the recipe) Sausage Balls, unshaped and uncooked, or migraine-safe, fresh bulk chicken sausage from a local butcher

½ cup trimmed, washed, and diced leeks (white and pale-green parts only)

7 large eggs

⅓ cup milk

1 teaspoon kosher salt

½ teaspoon ground sage

½ teaspoon dried marjoram

½ teaspoon garlic powder

½ teaspoon freshly ground black pepper

4 ounces fresh goat cheese (chèvre)

Preheat the oven to 350°F. In a large, deep skillet, add the chopped potatoes and cover with 2 inches of water. Bring the potatoes to a boil over high heat and boil until tender, about 5 minutes. Drain the potatoes, dry them on paper towels, and set off to the side.

Wipe the skillet clean, add the olive oil, and place over medium heat. Add the Sausage Balls and leeks. Cook, stirring, until the sausage is cooked through and the leeks are soft, about 5 minutes.

Meanwhile, crack the eggs into a medium bowl and add the milk, salt, sage, marjoram, garlic powder, and pepper. Whisk until combined.

Grease an 8-by-10-inch casserole pan with a little extra olive oil, then add the cooked potatoes and the leek and chicken mixture. Pour in the egg mixture, then crumble the goat cheese over the top. Place in the oven and bake until the eggs are set all the way through, 30 to 38 minutes. Cut into squares and serve warm.

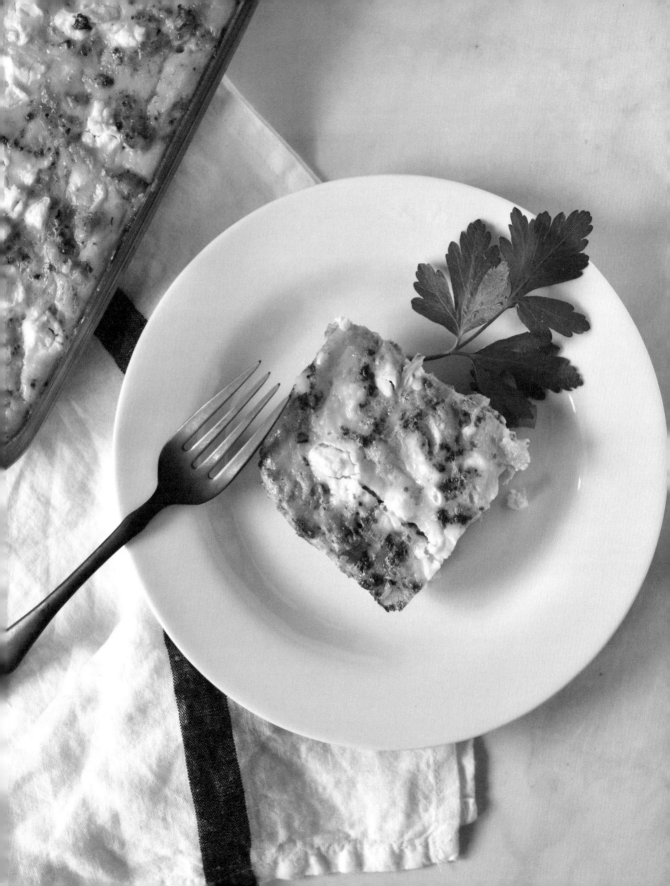

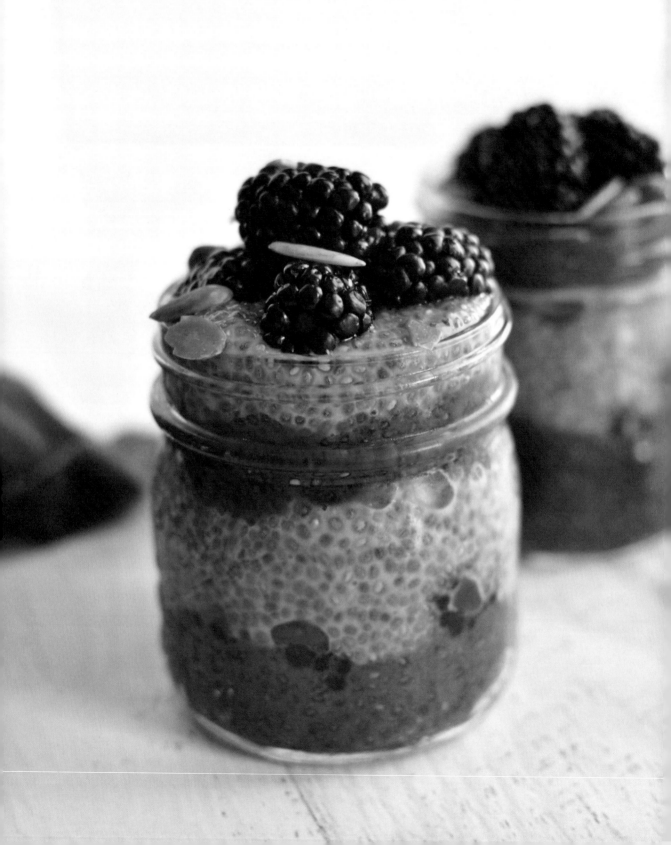

Blueberry & Vanilla Chia Pudding Parfait

MAKES 2 SERVINGS

Yogurt with berries was my go-to almost every morning when I was first diagnosed with vestibular migraine. But what I didn't realize before my migraine elimination diet was that yogurt was a huge trigger for me. Since I was in a chronic cycle at the time, I could never tell that it was increasing my symptoms. After I figured it out, I missed the simplicity of that breakfast. In an effort to find something similar, I tried multiple variations of chia pudding. The ratio below is my absolute favorite—not too mushy, just right. Chia is packed with fiber, which helps prevent rapid fluctuations in blood sugar. Combine this with a scoop of sunflower seed butter or a generous splash of homemade hemp milk (see sidebar on page 41), and you have a decent amount of protein as well. I love how fun these are layered together, but if it's too much work, they're also both delicious on their own.

VANILLA CHIA PUDDING

1 cup milk of choice

¼ cup chia seeds

2 teaspoons vanilla extract

2 teaspoons honey
   or maple syrup

BLUEBERRY CHIA PUDDING

½ cup frozen blueberries

¾ cup milk of choice

¼ cup chia seeds

2 teaspoons vanilla extract

TOPPINGS OF CHOICE

Hemp seeds

Pepitas (pumpkin seeds)

Sunflower seeds

Sunflower seed butter

Crunchy Buckwheat Granola
   (see page 45)

Blackberries

Blueberries

Peaches

Strawberries

Pomegranate seeds

To make the Vanilla Chia Pudding, add the milk, chia seeds, vanilla, and honey or maple syrup to a container, cover, and shake everything together well. Refrigerate for about 30 minutes, then stir well. Cover again and chill for 1 to 2 hours or overnight. Note: It is important you do not blend the chia seeds, or the pudding will become too gelatinous.

To make the Blueberry Chia Pudding, place the blueberries and milk in a blender and blend until fully combined. Pour the blueberry-milk mixture into a container along with the chia seeds and vanilla. Cover and shake everything together well. Refrigerate for about 30 minutes, then stir well. Cover again and chill for 1 to 2 hours or overnight. Note: It is important you do not blend the chia seeds, or the pudding will become too gelatinous.

Once the puddings have firmed up, layer each flavor in a clear bowl or parfait glass. Add any toppings you would like and enjoy!

Baked Bean Taquitos

MAKES 6 TAQUITOS

Coming up with breakfast recipes that provide a decent amount of protein without eggs can be a challenge. While eggs are allowed on a migraine diet, some sufferers find them to be a trigger. Frankly, I just get tired of them. I was trying to think of a substitute for breakfast tacos when the idea of using beans came to mind. There are few types of beans that are allowed on this migraine diet, including pinto and black. One cup will typically yield around 15 grams of protein. Looking at food a little bit differently can help us get out of the rut of eating the same thing every day on a restricted diet. Some other creative fillings for these taquitos are scrambled eggs or breakfast potatoes. These would also make a great snack or appetizer.

---

1 tablespoon olive oil, plus more for brushing tortillas

1 small shallot, finely chopped

⅓ cup finely chopped red bell pepper

1 (14-ounce) can pinto or black beans, drained

½ cup fresh spinach leaves

1 teaspoon distilled white vinegar

½ teaspoon garlic powder

½ teaspoon kosher salt

¼ teaspoon smoked paprika

5–6 flour or corn tortillas (TortillaLand is a safe brand and widely available)

Preheat oven to 425°F.

In a large skillet, warm 1 tablespoon olive oil over medium heat. Add the shallot and bell pepper and sauté until softened, about 2 minutes. Add the beans, spinach, vinegar, garlic powder, salt, and paprika. Continue cooking until the spinach has softened, about 3 minutes. Remove from heat. Mash the beans with the back of a spoon.

Lay out the tortillas in a single layer on a baking sheet. Divide the bean mixture among the tortillas, placing in a strip down the middle. Roll the tortillas tightly around the filling, then place them seam side down on the sheet to secure the filling. Brush the tops with a little more olive oil. Bake until the tortillas are light brown and crispy, about 20 minutes. Serve warm.

If you have any leftover taquitos, wrap them in foil and store in the refrigerator for up to 2 days. To reheat from the fridge, I place them on a baking sheet in the oven and turn it to 400°F. Once the oven reaches that temperature, I give them another 3 minutes. They should crisp up again nicely.

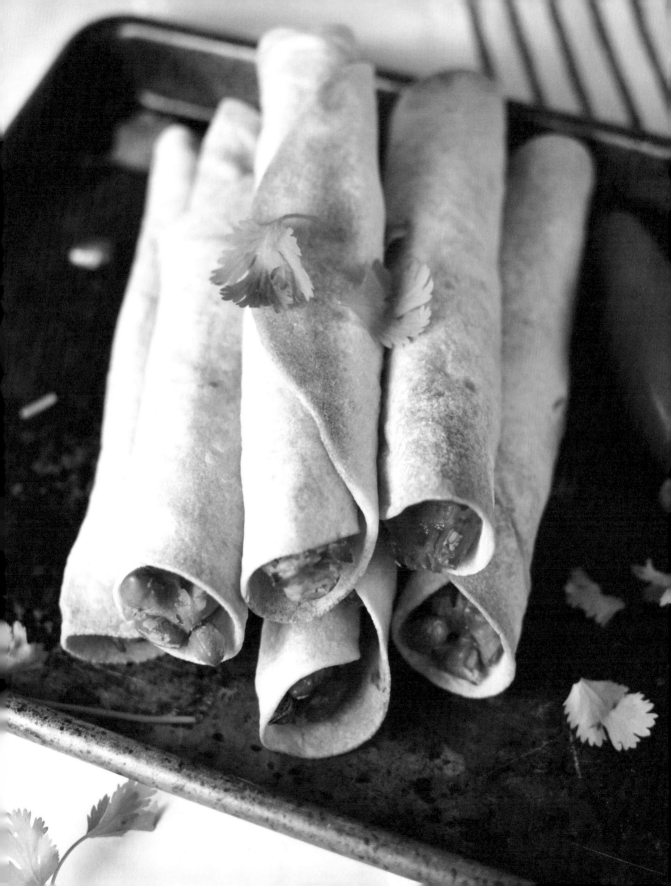

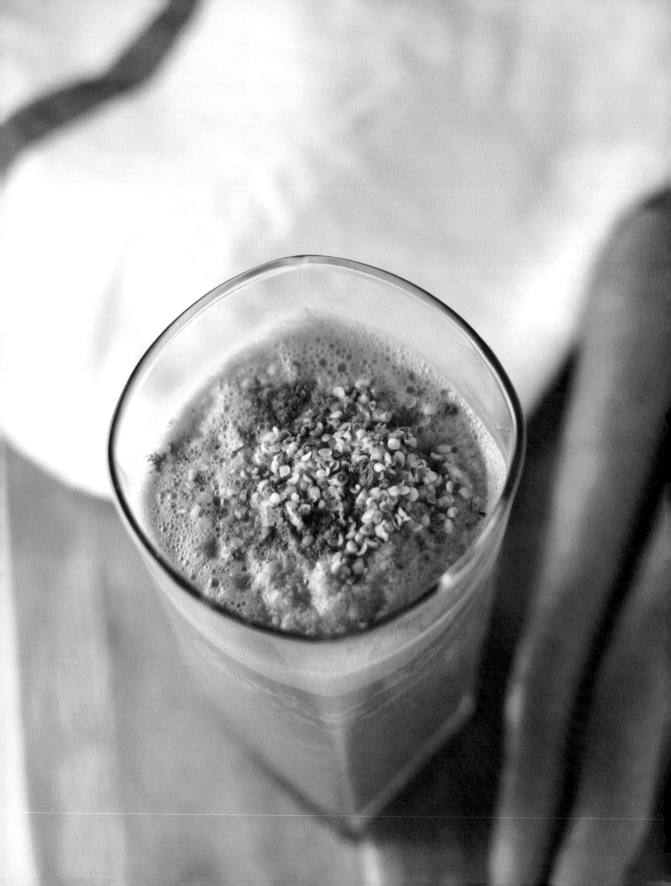

Carrot Spice Smoothie

MAKES 1 SERVING

You would not believe how good carrot juice is in a smoothie. It's sweet and sort of reminds me of fall… or perhaps that's just the spices I'm using. Either way, I promise you'll be blown away by the flavor. Carrot juice is easy to find at most health food stores, although I find the best deal is at Trader Joe's. You can find mini bottles in the refrigerator case there, which are perfect for this recipe. Carrots are packed with antioxidants, but the real star here is ginger, which is a powerful natural treatment that can effectively lower or eliminate migraine pain.

¾ cup fresh carrot juice

1 tablespoon sunflower seed butter or toasted sunflower seeds

1 tablespoon hemp seeds, plus more for garnish

1 teaspoon vanilla extract

½ teaspoon ground ginger

¼ teaspoon ground cinnamon

Ice cubes, as needed

Combine the carrot juice, sunflower seed butter, hemp seeds, vanilla, ginger, and cinnamon in a blender and blend on high until combined. Add ½ cup of ice at a time until the desired thickness is reached.

Pour into a tall glass, sprinkle with additional hemp seeds, and enjoy.

SB&J Smoothie

MAKES 1 SERVING

Peanut butter and jelly are one of the greatest flavor combinations known to humankind. A little sweetness mixed with savory, it was my go-to sandwich when I was an intern in NYC and could not afford much else. I wanted to capture that taste in a smoothie, but without the use of peanuts (a no-no because they can be a trigger like other legumes and nuts) or jelly (which is sometimes allowed depending on what kind you buy). Thankfully sunflower seed butter makes a wonderful substitute for peanut butter… have I sold you on sunflower seed butter yet?! I like to use hemp milk for this recipe to boost the protein content, but any milk you like will do. I prefer the taste and texture of frozen wild blueberries to fresh for this recipe, but any frozen blueberries will work.

¾ cup frozen blueberries, preferably wild, plus more for garnish

¾ cup milk of choice, preferably hemp

2 tablespoons sunflower seed butter or toasted sunflower seeds

½ teaspoon vanilla extract

2 tablespoons dried mulberries, for sweetening, plus more for garnish (optional)

About ½ cup of ice

Combine the blueberries, milk, sunflower seed butter, vanilla, and mulberries, if using, in a blender and slowly increase the speed until everything is blended smoothly. Add the ice and continue to blend until smooth.

Pour into a tall glass, garnish with additional dried mulberries and blueberries, if desired, and enjoy.

SUNFLOWER SEED BUTTER The key to this smoothie—and to many migraine-safe recipes in this book—is finding a brand of sunflower seed butter you really love. There are many different flavor combinations out there. Some are salted, some have extra sugar, some are flavored with vanilla and cinnamon. I personally prefer the slightly salted, unsweetened version for this recipe.

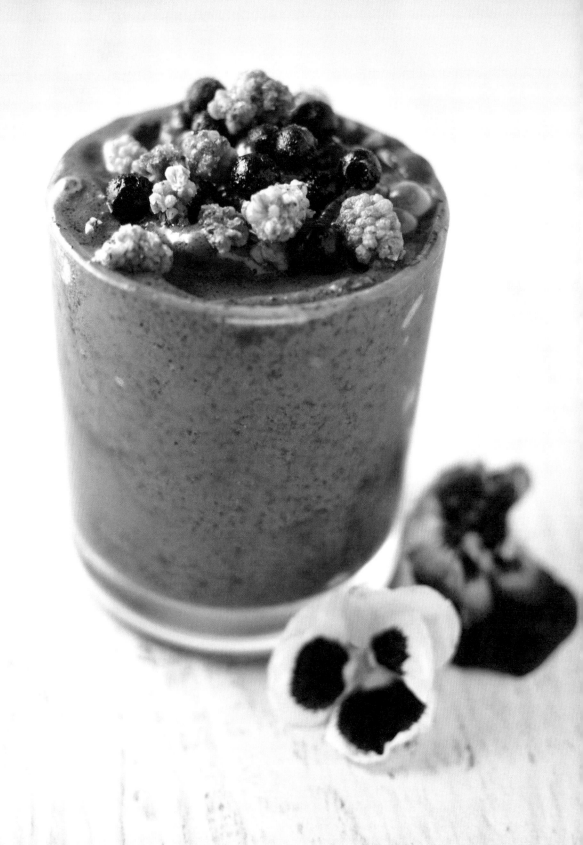

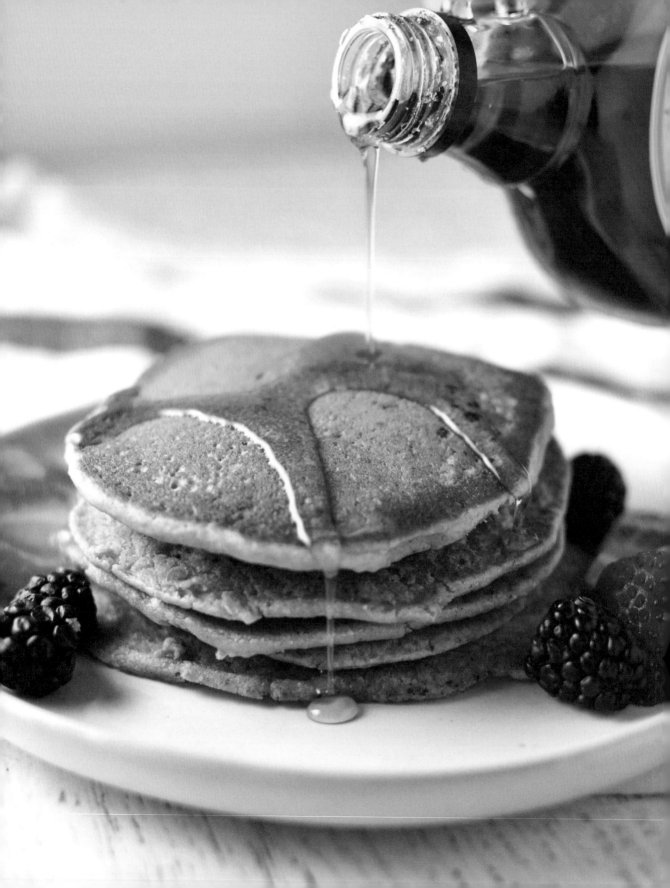

Nutty Pancakes

MAKES 8 PANCAKES

I had to laugh at this recipe name knowing all of us can relate to feeling a bit nutty when we get an attack. Nutmeg is a ground seed whose flavor brings back memories of oatmeal cookies and pumpkin spice lattes from my teenage years when I needed to add five gallons of sugar to drink any amount of coffee. Actually, that's how I got the idea for this recipe—I wanted it to taste like those delicious oatmeal cookies of my past. Fortunately, these pancakes are much healthier. They have a strong nutmeg flavor, so if you're not a fan, consider reducing it to ¼ teaspoon or replacing with cinnamon. To make oat flour at home, pulse rolled oats in a food processor until they are finely ground and powdery. I would use 1¾ cups of oats to make sure you have plenty for this recipe.

1¼ cups oat flour (certified gluten-free, if desired)

2 teaspoons baking powder

½ teaspoon ground nutmeg

¾ cup milk of choice

¼ cup applesauce

1 tablespoon unsalted butter, melted, or neutral oil

1 tablespoon honey or maple syrup

1 teaspoon vanilla extract

1 teaspoon distilled white vinegar

¼ teaspoon kosher salt

Neutral oil for cooking

OPTIONAL TOPPINGS

Maple syrup

Sunflower seed butter

Sliced or whole migraine-friendly fruit of choice

In a large bowl, combine the oat flour, baking powder, and nutmeg. In another bowl, combine the milk, applesauce, butter or oil, honey or maple syrup, vanilla, vinegar, and salt, and mix well. Make a well in the flour mixture and pour the milk-applesauce mixture into the well. Mix until smooth.

Heat a lightly oiled griddle or skillet over medium heat. To form each pancake, using a ¼-cup scoop, pour the batter onto the hot griddle and leave it alone until it's bubbling at the top and set on the sides. (The biggest mistake you can make with these pancakes is flipping them too early, because they will crumble.) Brown on the opposite side. Keep the pancakes warm by covering under tin foil while you cook the remaining pancakes. Serve immediately with the toppings of your choice.

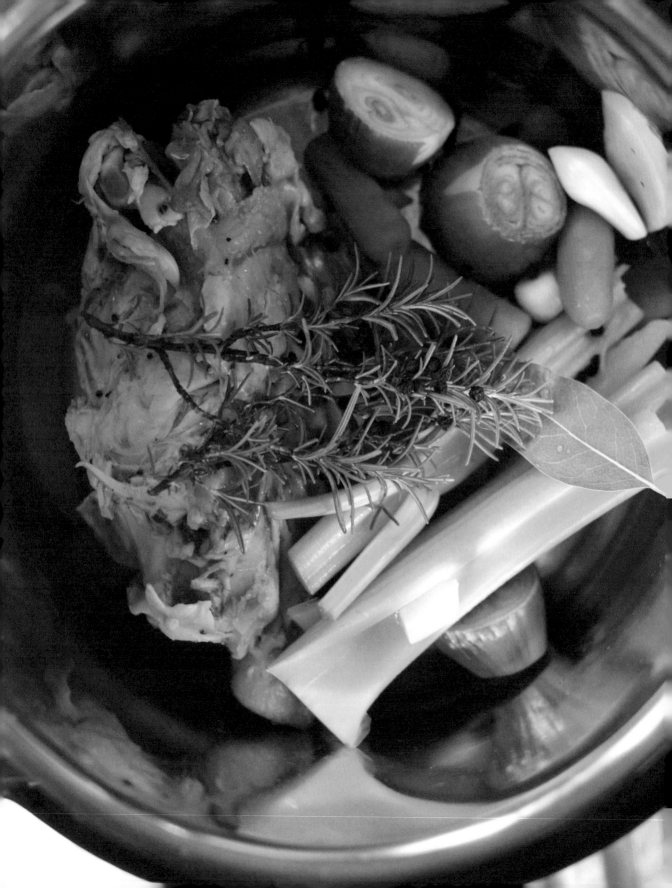

Kitchen Basics: Dressings, Condiments, Broth & Stock

I'm a strong believer that the perfect condiment or sauce can elevate any meal. We do it all the time for Thanksgiving. Bland turkey? Cover it in tons of gravy! However, condiments can be one of the biggest stressors on a migraine diet. It's next to impossible to find store-bought dressings that don't contain some form of tyramine, aged vinegar, hidden MSG, or other additives. And most stocks and broths contain "natural flavors" or "yeast extract"—alternative names for monosodium glutamate. Plus, anything packaged is not exactly fresh, and that's our number-one rule with this diet.

The following pages feature eleven recipes for condiments that are migraine-friendly, so you won't have to worry about finding safe store-bought versions. The good news is that you can make most of these recipes quickly, and they often taste better than any purchased brand you might find.

These dressings taste more flavorful the longer the flavors have time to combine. I typically keep them for up to three to four days, as tyramine buildup is less of an issue if there's not much protein. That said, if you know you're generally sensitive to leftovers, cut the recipe in half so you can use it quickly. A note about oils: Most people with migraine disease find they tolerate all kinds very well. This is because oils are highly refined and less likely to trigger. It's similar to why certain people with peanut allergies can tolerate peanut oil.

As for mayonnaise, there are not many store-bought versions that are totally "safe." My favorite is Sir Kensington's Organic, which has a minuscule amount of lemon juice. I figure it's much better than the others with a long list of ingredients I can't pronounce. Making your own is also very easy. There are many recipes online—just make sure to substitute distilled white vinegar for lemon juice. I have recipes for migraine-friendly mayos (traditional and vegan) at thedizzycook.com.

I use Dijon mustard in some of these recipes (and throughout the book). It can be tricky since many versions contain wine and sulfites. Look for brands that do not contain these triggers, like Annie's Organic.

Honey Mustard Dressing

MAKES ABOUT ¾ CUP

A total crowd-pleaser, this dressing is a healthier update to the traditional mayo-packed version. It's wonderful tossed with kale and spinach for a simple salad. I also love to add a hardboiled egg, thinly sliced shallot, tomatoes, homemade croutons, and cucumbers for a big lunch.

½ cup extra-virgin olive oil or neutral oil

¼ cup *each* honey and Dijon mustard (wine- and sulfite-free)

2 tablespoons distilled white vinegar

1 tablespoon apple juice

½ clove garlic, minced

½ teaspoon kosher salt

¼ teaspoon freshly ground black pepper

In a bowl, combine the oil, honey, mustard, vinegar, apple juice, garlic, salt, and pepper. Whisk all the ingredients together until smooth and creamy. Use right away or transfer to a storage container and refrigerate until ready to use (within 3 to 4 days).

Ginger Sesame Dressing

MAKES ABOUT ½ CUP

Slightly sweet and tangy, this Asian-inspired dressing is perfect when tossed with mixed greens, cucumber, and carrots. It can be drizzled over seared fish, especially ahi tuna, and brown rice. It's also great tossed with cabbage as a slaw or added to rice noodles for lunch or dinner.

2 tablespoons *each* neutral oil, toasted sesame oil, and pear juice

1 tablespoon distilled white vinegar

1 tablespoon tahini

2 teaspoons minced fresh ginger

1 clove garlic, minced

½ teaspoon kosher salt

In a small bowl, combine the neutral oil, sesame oil, pear juice, vinegar, tahini, ginger, garlic, and salt. Whisk everything together until smooth and chill for 30 minutes. Use right away or transfer to a storage container and refrigerate until ready to use (within 3 to 4 days).

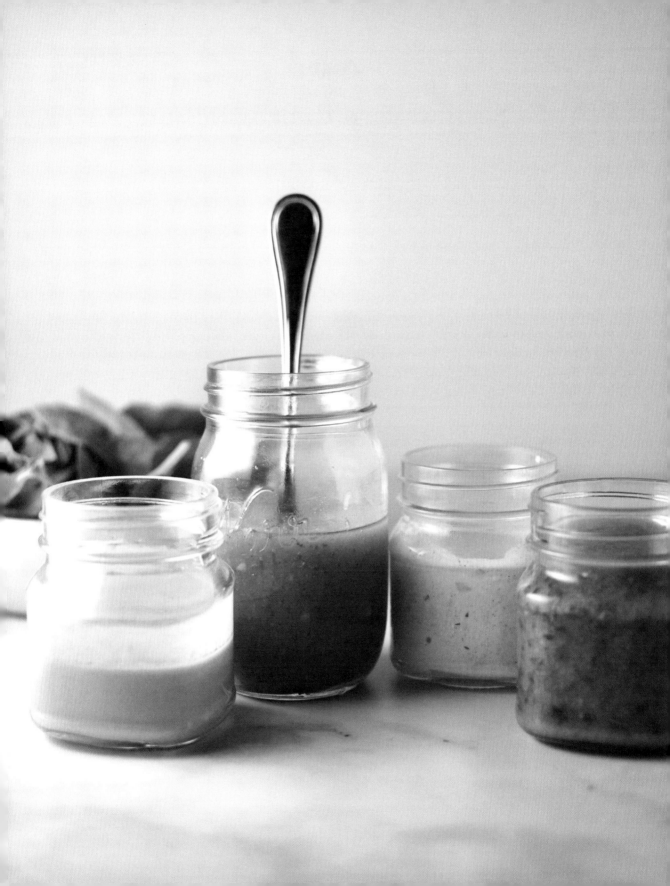

Southwestern Ranch Dressing

MAKES ABOUT ½ CUP

A flavorful take on traditional ranch, this version is great on taco salads or with barbecue-style dishes. If you're looking for a more classic ranch flavor, replace the smoked paprika with regular paprika and the cumin with dried dill.

¼ cup milk of choice

⅓ cup migraine-friendly mayonnaise

1 teaspoon distilled white vinegar

1 tablespoon chopped fresh parsley

½ teaspoon *each* kosher salt and garlic powder

¼ teaspoon *each* ground cumin and smoked paprika

In a bowl, whisk together the milk, mayonnaise, vinegar, parsley, salt, garlic powder, cumin, and smoked paprika. Chill for 30 minutes. The dressing will thicken as it chills, but I find it to be less thick when using dairy milk alternatives like oat or hemp milk. Use right away or transfer to a storage container and refrigerate until ready to use (within 3 to 4 days).

Italian Dressing

MAKES ABOUT 1¼ CUPS

I'm a huge fan of any dressing with lots of fresh herbs, and this one hits the spot. I make a big batch of this on Sunday and use it on side salads throughout the week. It's especially tasty on butter lettuce or romaine with some chopped carrots and cucumber.

¾ cup extra-virgin olive oil

¼ cup distilled white vinegar

1 cup loosely packed fresh Italian parsley

⅓ cup fresh basil

1 clove garlic, peeled

1 teaspoon honey

¾ teaspoon kosher salt

½ teaspoon dried oregano

¼ teaspoon freshly ground black pepper

In a food processor, combine the olive oil, vinegar, parsley, basil, garlic, honey, salt, oregano, and pepper. Process until smooth. Use right away or transfer to a storage container and refrigerate until ready to use (within 3 to 4 days).

1-2-3 Dressing
(a.k.a. The Easiest Dressing in the World)

MAKES ABOUT ⅓ CUP

If you're new to cooking, this will be the holy grail of dressings. This is one that my grandma taught my mom, who eventually passed it on to me. It's quick and easy and can even be made without any measuring. It's based on a simple ratio, so you can scale it up or down easily, depending on how many servings you need. You can play around with this base, adding whatever herbs and spices you like. Some minced fresh garlic and Dijon mustard is great whisked in too. The options are limitless! (Well, except for aged vinegars and onion.)

---

3 tablespoons oil, such as extra-virgin olive oil or neutral oil

2 tablespoons distilled white vinegar

1 tablespoon sweetener, such as honey or maple syrup

Kosher salt and freshly ground black pepper

Put the oil, vinegar, and sweetener in a bowl and whisk until well blended. Adjust the proportions to your own personal taste. Season to taste with salt and pepper. Use right away or transfer to a storage container and refrigerate until ready to use (within 3 to 4 days).

SALAD DRESSING STORAGE I like to use a Mason jar for my dressings for easy storage. To ensure there's no tyramine buildup, I store my dressings in the refrigerator for three to four days, but don't be surprised if the ones with olive oil get clumpy. Olive oil can firm up in the fridge, so just leave it out at room temperature for a few minutes and whisk again before serving.

Celery Seed Dressing

MAKES ABOUT ⅔ CUP

The second I knew I was creating a cookbook, I asked my grandma (who is now ninety-six years old and still cooking every day) for a few of my favorite recipes of hers. One of them is this celery seed dressing. When I saw that it contained ½ cup of white sugar, I knew I had to edit it a bit to make this a little more migraine friendly. So, here's the healthy-ish version of Grandma Mary's famous celery seed dressing. You can find celery seed in the spice aisle of your local grocery store. Use it for simple side salads, or I love to toss it with greens and top with Pepita-Poppyseed Chicken Salad (see page 94) for lunch.

½ cup neutral oil

3 tablespoons honey
or maple syrup

2 tablespoons distilled white
vinegar

1 tablespoon apple juice

1 small shallot, minced

¾ teaspoon celery seed

½ teaspoon kosher salt

¼ teaspoon dry mustard

In a bowl, combine the oil, honey or maple syrup, vinegar, apple juice, shallot, celery seed, salt, and dry mustard. Whisk all the ingredients together until thoroughly combined. Use right away or transfer to a storage container and refrigerate until ready to use (within 3 to 4 days).

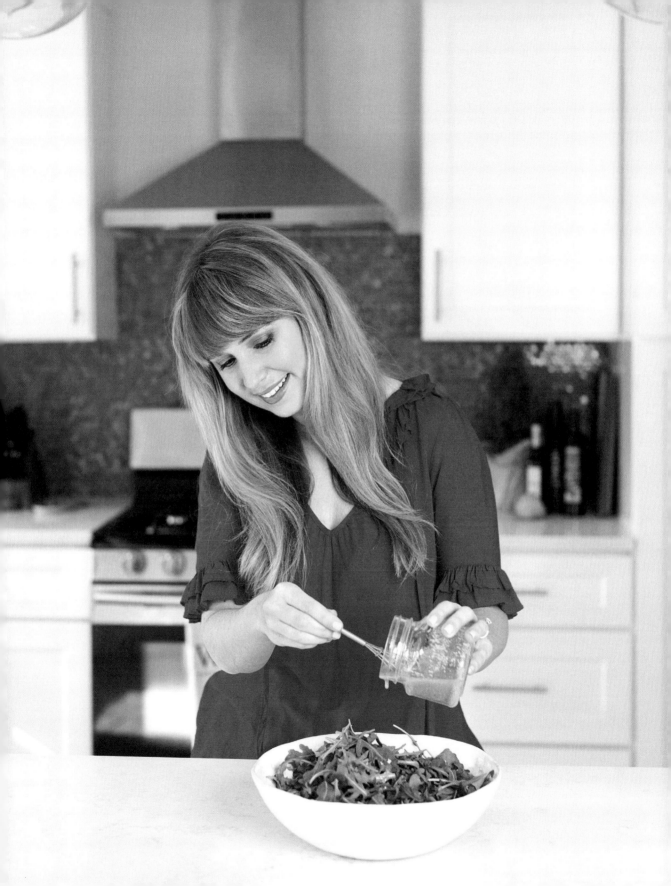

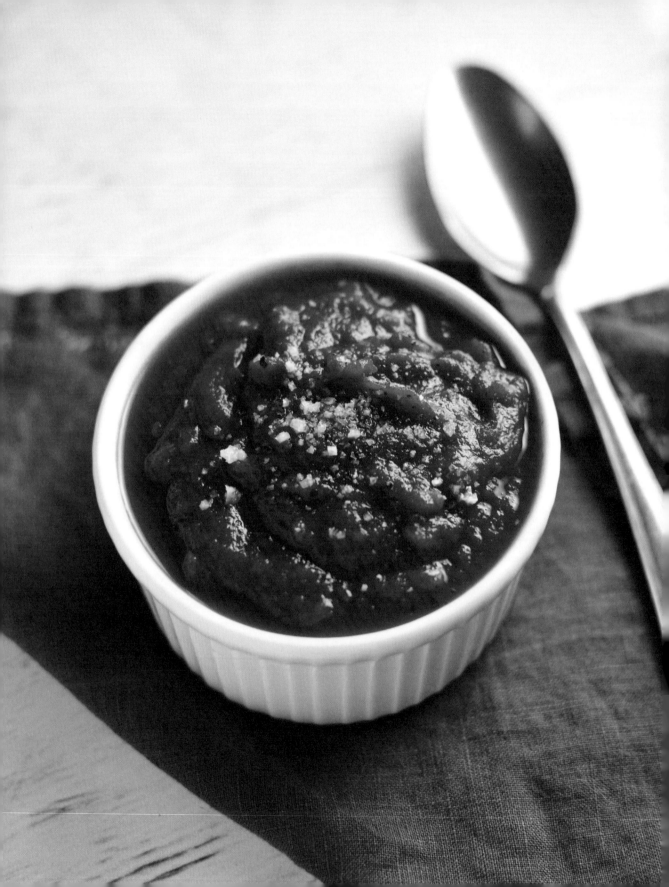

Barbecue Sauce

MAKES ABOUT 1½ CUPS

This is one recipe that I am beyond proud of. I have not found any good barbecue sauce recipes out there that don't use some kind of fake smoke flavor or migraine-triggering ingredients. Trust me, I've looked. I originally tested this recipe out on the Mini Barbecue Meatloaves (page 146), but since then I've made it multiple times for pulled pork, burgers, and chicken. Strained tomatoes are basically pureed tomatoes without excess moisture, seeds, and skin. Make sure to check the label on the tomatoes—they should only contain one or two ingredients, and one of them should be tomatoes.

2 tablespoons minced shallot

1 large clove garlic, minced

2 tablespoons apple juice

13 ounces (1½ cups) strained tomatoes (Pomì is a good brand)

1½ tablespoons light brown sugar

2 teaspoons smoked paprika

½ teaspoon dry mustard

⅛ teaspoon cayenne pepper

Kosher salt to taste

In a small saucepan, combine the shallot, garlic, and apple juice. Cook over medium heat, stirring often, until the shallots and garlic are fragrant and softened, about 1 minute. Add the tomatoes, brown sugar, smoked paprika, dry mustard, and cayenne. Bring to a simmer. Reduce heat to low and cook for 20 minutes, stirring frequently. Add kosher salt to taste.

Remove the sauce from the heat and allow to cool and let the flavors meld for about 30 minutes. Use right away or transfer to a storage container and refrigerate until ready to use (within 3 to 4 days) or freeze for up to 3 months.

Pepita Pesto

MAKES ABOUT ¾ CUP

About as fun to eat as it is to say, you won't miss Parmesan cheese or nuts in this glorious pesto. It uses toasted pepitas (pumpkin seeds), mixed herbs, and greens. I've tried this recipe with both sunflower seeds and pepitas, and I personally prefer the pepitas, but feel free to use whatever you have on hand. This is wonderful on flatbreads as a sauce, tossed with pasta, and served as a dip for chicken or vegetables.

⅓ cup raw pepitas (pumpkin seeds)

1 clove garlic

1 cup fresh spinach

1 cup fresh basil

1 cup arugula

⅓ cup extra-virgin olive oil

2 teaspoons distilled white vinegar

¼ teaspoon kosher salt, or more to taste

Freshly ground black pepper to taste

To toast the pepitas, place them in a dry pan and cook over medium-low heat, stirring often, until lightly toasted, 3 to 4 minutes total. Transfer to a food processor and let cool.

Add the garlic to the processor with the pepitas and process until the mixture resembles sand. Add the spinach, basil, and arugula and process again until finely chopped. Add the olive oil, vinegar, and salt; process until fairly smooth. Add more salt and pepper to taste. Use right away or transfer to a storage container and refrigerate until ready to use (within 3 to 4 days) or freeze for up to 3 months.

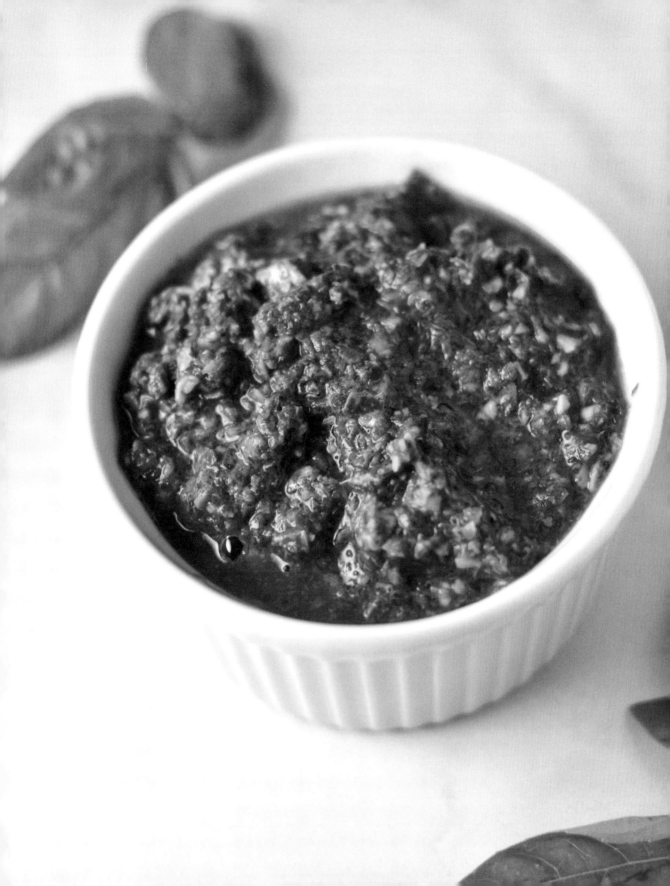

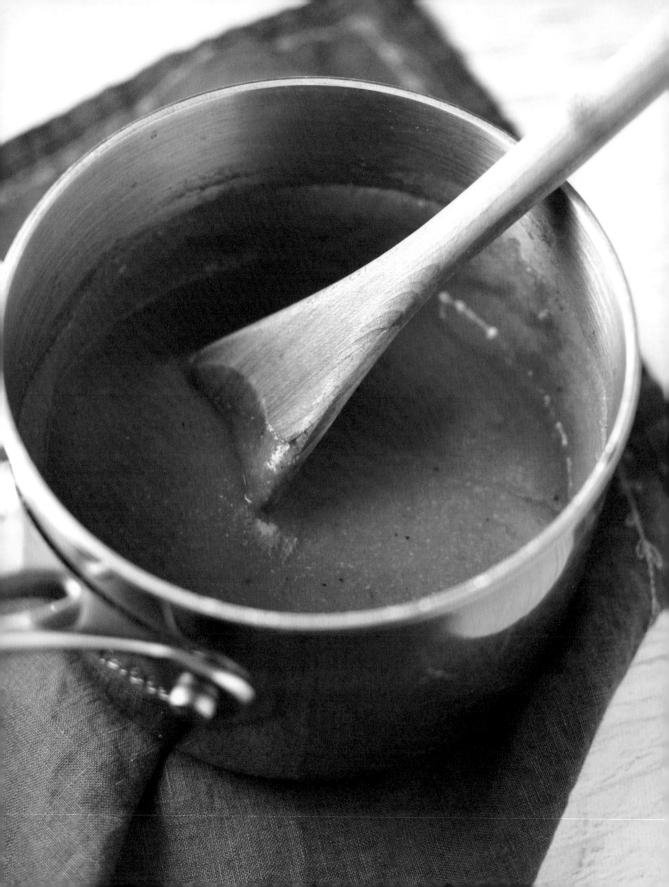

Enchilada Sauce

MAKES ABOUT 1¼ CUPS

Once you make your own enchilada sauce, you'll wonder why you haven't been doing it all along. It's beyond easy and uses basic pantry ingredients, plus it doesn't contain any MSG like many canned sauces do. I use it in the Mexican-Style Stuffed Sweet Potatoes (page 145) and for chicken, beef, and/or vegetable enchiladas. If you have trouble with tomatoes, just leave the tomato paste out of the recipe. It's still delicious without it.

3 tablespoons extra-virgin olive oil

3 tablespoons all-purpose flour, sweet rice flour, or white rice flour

1 tablespoon tomato paste

1 tablespoon chili powder

1 teaspoon ground cumin

1 teaspoon garlic powder

1 teaspoon kosher salt

1½ cups Vegetable Broth (page 80) or Chicken Stock (page 81)

1 teaspoon distilled white vinegar

In a small saucepan, combine the olive oil and flour over medium heat, whisking until smooth. Add the tomato paste, chili powder, cumin, garlic powder, and salt, and cook, stirring continuously, until fragrant, about 1 minute. Whisk in the broth or stock until smooth, and simmer over medium heat until slightly reduced and thickened, 4 to 5 minutes. Turn off the heat and stir in the vinegar. The sauce will thicken as it cools.

Use right away or transfer to a storage container and refrigerate until ready to use (within 3 to 4 days).

Vegetable Broth
MAKES ABOUT 2 QUARTS

I only used my Instant Pot occasionally until I began making my own stocks and broths—now I use it constantly! It saves so much time and it's amazing for those who are sensitive to tyramine buildup from stocks simmered all day long. What I never realized until following a migraine diet is that most store-bought stocks and broths are filled with "natural chicken flavor" or "yeast extract," which are hidden names for monosodium glutamate. I also have yet to find one without onion as an ingredient.

---

1 tablespoon extra-virgin olive oil

5 cloves garlic, smashed and peeled

4 large carrots, roughly chopped

4 celery stalks, roughly chopped

2 leeks, trimmed, cut in half, and roughly chopped (white and pale-green parts only)

2 bay leaves

1 tablespoon black peppercorns

1 tablespoon distilled white vinegar

2 teaspoons kosher salt

Handful of fresh parsley, thyme, and rosemary

9–10 cups of water

Turn the Instant Pot to "Sauté." When the pot is hot, add the olive oil, garlic, carrots, celery, and leeks. Sauté the vegetables until soft and fragrant, 3 to 5 minutes. Add the bay leaves, peppercorns, vinegar, salt, and herbs, then pour the water into the pot, being careful not to exceed the pot's fill line.

Following the manufacturer's instructions, secure the lid and close the steam release valve, then press the "Pressure Cook" button and set the timer for 30 minutes. The pressure will build, and the lid should seal within 10 to 15 minutes.

Once the timer finishes, allow a natural release; do not touch the lid or release valve for another 15 minutes. When the 15 minutes are up, follow the manufacturer's instructions to carefully open the release valve to let any remaining steam escape. Remove the lid.

To make this in a slow cooker, follow the same instructions but cook on high for 4 hours or on low for 8 hours. To make this on the stovetop, simmer for 2 to 4 hours.

Pour the broth through a fine-mesh sieve into a heatproof bowl. Discard solids and let the broth cool completely.

Store the broth in Mason jars (use within 2 days) or in locking plastic bags that you can lay flat in the freezer. Pouring into ice cube trays and freezing is perfect for individual portions.

Chicken Stock

MAKES ABOUT 2 QUARTS

I use my Instant Pot for this recipe too. I love to get a "naked" rotisserie chicken from the store, pick off the meat and freeze it for lunches that week, then use the bones to make a big batch of chicken stock. If you're not ready to make this right away, freeze the chicken carcass until ready to use.

1 cooked chicken carcass, picked of meat

3 celery stalks, roughly chopped

3 large carrots, roughly chopped

4 cloves garlic, smashed and peeled

1 shallot, peeled and halved

3 sprigs thyme

3 sprigs rosemary

1 bay leaf

1 tablespoon black peppercorns

1 teaspoon kosher salt

9–10 cups of water

Add the chicken carcass, celery, carrots, garlic, shallot, thyme, rosemary, bay leaf, peppercorns, and salt to the Instant Pot. Put the water into the pot, being careful not to exceed the pot's fill line. Following the manufacturer's instructions, secure the lid and close the steam release valve, then press the "Pressure Cook" button and set the timer for 40 minutes. The pressure will build, and the lid should seal within 10 to 15 minutes.

Once the timer finishes, allow a natural release; do not touch the lid or release valve for another 15 minutes. When the 15 minutes are up, follow the manufacturer's instructions to carefully open the release valve to let any remaining steam escape. Remove the lid.

To make this in a slow cooker, follow the same instructions but cook on high for 4 hours or on low for 8 hours. To make this on the stovetop, simmer for 2 to 4 hours.

Pour the broth through a fine-mesh sieve into a heatproof bowl. Discard solids and let the broth cool completely.

Store the broth in Mason jars (use within 2 days) or in locking plastic bags that you can lay flat in the freezer. Pouring into ice cube trays and freezing is perfect for individual portions.

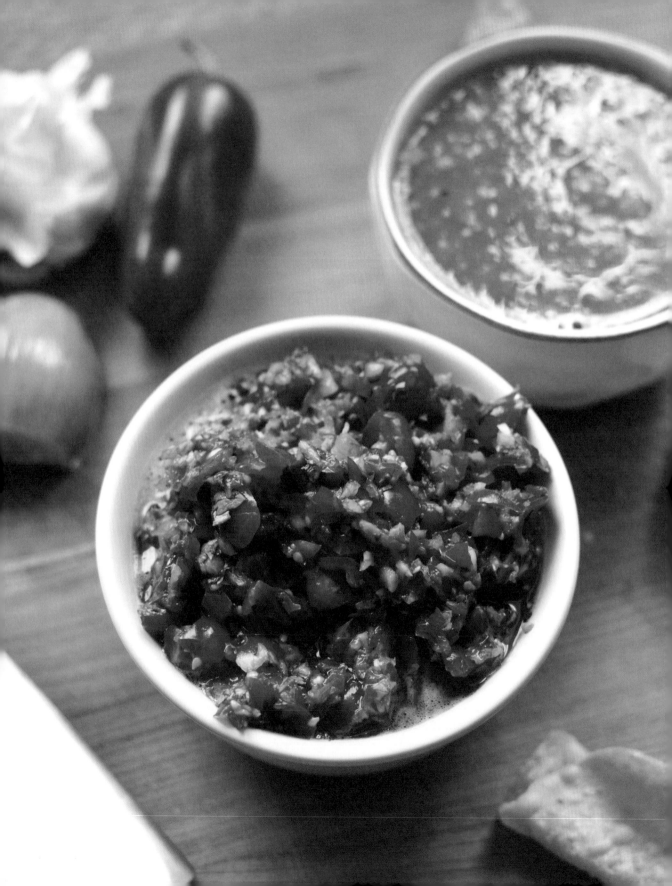

A Tale of Two Salsas

MAKES ABOUT 1 CUP EACH

Occasionally, I'll find a salsa verde out there that's migraine safe, but I also live in Texas, so I recognize that my salsa options are slightly more plentiful here than in other parts of the country. Here are two quick recipes that you can whip up for nachos, tacos, enchiladas, and more.

QUICK TOMATO SALSA

1 small shallot, peeled

1 clove garlic, peeled

⅓ cup fresh cilantro

2 teaspoons distilled white vinegar

1 pint cherry tomatoes

Kosher salt and freshly ground black pepper

CHARRED SALSA VERDE

4–6 large tomatillos, about 1 pound total

1 shallot, peeled

2 cloves garlic, unpeeled

½ small jalapeño, seeds and ribs removed for less heat (optional)

¼ cup fresh cilantro

Kosher salt to taste

To make the Quick Tomato Salsa, in a small food processor, combine the shallot, garlic, cilantro, and vinegar, and pulse until finely chopped. Add the cherry tomatoes and pulse until the salsa is the consistency you prefer. Add salt and pepper to taste. Transfer to a small serving bowl and allow to sit at room temperature for about 30 minutes. Serve, or refrigerate in an airtight container and use within 2 to 3 days.

To make the Charred Salsa Verde, position the oven rack in the middle-upper position (about 6 inches from the heat source) and set the broiler to high. Meanwhile, peel the papery skin from the tomatillos and run them under warm water to clean off some of the stickiness. Transfer to a baking sheet. Add the shallot, garlic, and jalapeño (if using).

Place the baking sheet under the broiler and set the timer for 5 minutes, or until black splotches begin to appear on the vegetables. Use tongs to flip the tomatillos and shallots to char on the opposite side and remove garlic and jalapeño if they are already covered in dark spots. Then broil the flipped tomatillos and shallots for an additional 5 minutes, or until they are charred all over. Transfer sheet to a wire rack to cool.

When garlic is cool enough to handle, remove the skins and add the peeled garlic to a blender or food processor. Add the remaining contents of the baking sheet (including juices) to the blender along with the cilantro. Pulse until smooth. Add salt to taste and serve right away or refrigerate in an airtight container and use within 2 to 3 days. Warm for a few seconds in the microwave before serving again.

TOMATILLOS If you have trouble tolerating tomatoes, don't rule out tomatillos immediately. Tomatillos come from an entirely different plant, so while some people find they cannot tolerate tomatoes, they occasionally have better luck with tomatillos.

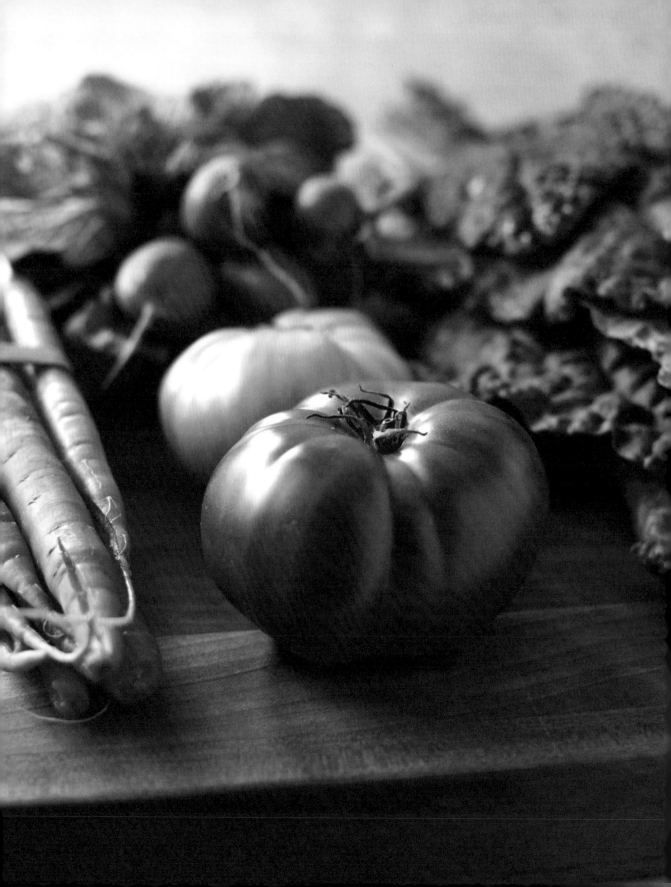

Salads & Soups

This will become your go-to chapter for those rough days where cooking just seems like an overwhelming task. These salads are easy to prepare and most of the ingredients are pantry staples. They make tasty lunches as well as quick and easy dinners. One of my favorites, the Mediterranean Pita Salad with Faux Tzatziki, can be transformed into a filling meal with the addition of simply grilled chicken or meatballs. And we never miss a Fourth of July without the Charred Corn & Farro Summer Salad. Don't skip the Chilled Soba Noodle Salad, which is the perfect riff on migraine-safe takeout at its finest.

As for these soups, the Farro & Lemongrass Chicken Soup is the perfect update to a traditional chicken noodle. I swear it has magical healing powers when you're struggling with a cold. And the Curried Carrot & Sweet Potato Soup has pain-fighting power, with ginger and turmeric. I like to freeze my soups in locking plastic bags so I can easily thaw individual portions on nights I don't feel up to cooking.

Maui Kale Salad

MAKES 4 TO 6 SIDE-DISH SERVINGS

My first long flight after being diagnosed with vestibular migraine was to Maui, about a year after my symptoms began. I was not only terrified of the flight triggering symptoms I was barely managing, I was also just a few months into the Heal Your Headache diet. I remember packing Seed Butter Energy Balls (page 131) and a kale salad for the flight since I knew the airplane food would not be migraine friendly. It wasn't the vacation dreams are made of, but we used miles to go back the next year and make all new memories. On my second trip, I survived a boat ride to do a sunrise snorkel and was proud of myself for taking a chance. Just two years before I felt like I was on a boat, and here I was on a boat… and enjoying it. This recipe is an ode to our Maui trips where I conquered many fears—and ate a lot of great kale salads. I love to switch out the cheese sometimes with fresh goat cheese (chèvre). If you want to skip all the greens prep, substitute the kale, cabbage, and Brussels sprouts with one 10-ounce bag of Trader Joe's Cruciferous Crunch Salad Mix.

⅓ cup raw sunflower seeds

1 bunch lacinato (dinosaur) kale

½ head *each* purple and green cabbage, or 3 cups pre-shredded purple and green cabbage mix

½ pound Brussels sprouts or 1 (8-ounce) package pre-shredded Brussels sprouts

1 green apple, sliced or chopped

½ cup chopped English cucumber

⅓ cup shredded good-quality white American cheese or crumbled fresh goat cheese (chèvre)

Honey Mustard Dressing (page 68)

½ cup dried cranberries (sulfite-free) or fresh pomegranate seeds

To toast the sunflower seeds, place them in a dry pan over medium-low heat. Toast them, tossing around every so often until lightly browned, 4 to 5 minutes. Transfer to a plate and let cool.

If you're not using pre-packaged mixes, wash the kale, cabbage, and sprouts and spin them dry. Remove the thick rib from each kale leaf, then stack the leaves and slice thinly. Remove the cores from the cabbage and thinly slice or shred on a mandoline. Remove the stems from the Brussels sprouts and thinly slice or shred on a mandoline.

Transfer vegetables to a large bowl. Add the apple, cucumber, and cheese, then toss with the dressing, using just enough for an even coating. Sprinkle with dried cranberries or pomegranate seeds and serve.

> **CHEESE TIP** To find a "good-quality American cheese" that is likely to be HYH compliant, look for brands in the fresh cheese area. Andrew & Everett and Boar's Head are good brands.

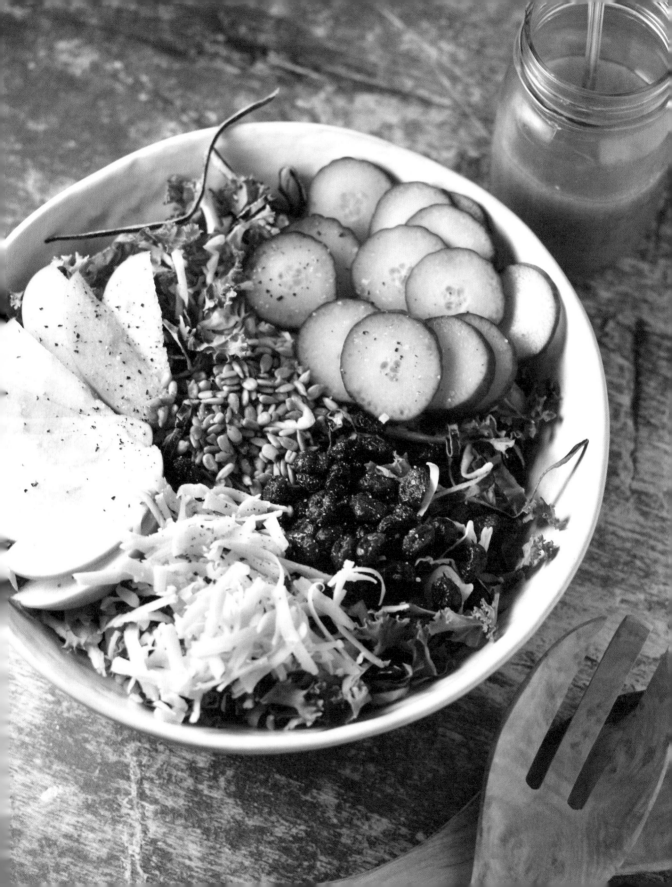

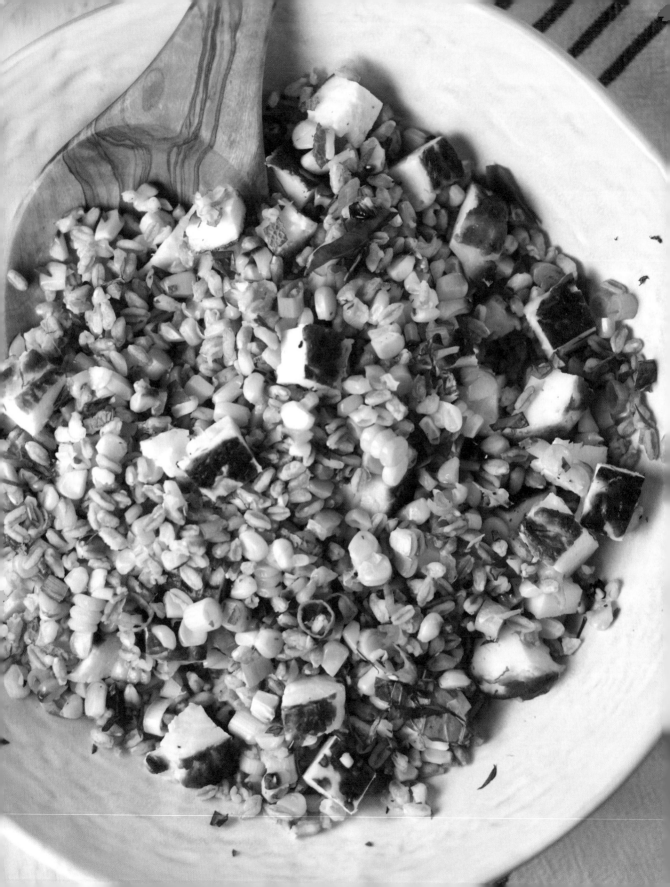

Charred Corn & Farro Summer Salad

MAKES 4 TO 6 SIDE-DISH SERVINGS

This is one salad that I make for every barbecue and Fourth of July. Halloumi is a fresh cheese that many people are not familiar with. Its texture is similar to mozzarella but slightly thicker, and it doesn't melt readily, making it perfect for sautéing, grilling, or broiling. You want to make sure you get the unaged kind. The only part that makes it slightly risky for migraine sufferers is that halloumi is brined. While many do tolerate it well, a great substitute if you are concerned, especially if you are just starting the HYH diet, is fresh mozzarella (unbroiled, of course).

---

1 cup pearled farro

½ cup raw pepitas (pumpkin seeds)

4 ears fresh yellow corn, shucked

1 tablespoon plus ¼ cup extra-virgin olive oil, divided

Kosher salt and freshly ground black pepper

1 (8-ounce) package halloumi or fresh mozzarella

3 green onions, chopped

2 tablespoons minced fresh parsley

2 tablespoons minced fresh basil

2 teaspoons minced fresh mint

2 tablespoons distilled white vinegar

Cook the farro according to package directions and set aside. To a dry small skillet, add the pepitas over medium-low heat, stirring often, until lightly toasted, 3 to 4 minutes total. Transfer to a plate to cool.

Position the oven rack in the top position and set the broiler to high. Place the corn ears on a baking sheet and rub with 1 tablespoon olive oil. Sprinkle with kosher salt and pepper. Broil the corn, turning it every 5 to 6 minutes, until there's a nice char on both sides, 10 to 12 minutes total. Remove the corn from the oven and allow to cool. (Leave on the broiler and reserve the baking sheet if using halloumi.) Remove the kernels and transfer to a large bowl.

If using halloumi, place the cheese on the baking sheet and broil until browned on each large side, 3 to 4 minutes per side. Allow the halloumi to cool, then cut it into cubes. If using mozzarella, just cut it into cubes without broiling (otherwise it would be a melted mess). Transfer cheese to the bowl with the corn.

To the large bowl with the corn and cheese, add green onions, parsley, basil, mint, vinegar, and the remaining ¼ cup olive oil, cooked farro, and toasted pepitas. Stir everything together until well combined. Add salt and pepper to taste before serving. (Halloumi is saltier than mozzarella, so adjust accordingly.)

Summer Pasta Salad with Zesty Herb Dressing

MAKES 4 TO 6 SIDE-DISH SERVINGS

Unlike traditional pasta salad, this version does not have mayonnaise. The fact that you can let it sit out for a while without worrying about spoiling makes it perfect for road trips where you're wary of fast food choices. It's also an ideal choice to bring to potlucks when you want a filling item in case there's not much else on offer that's migraine safe. I like to use quinoa pasta for a gluten-free option. Carrots can be substituted for cherry tomatoes if the latter are not well tolerated.

SUMMER PASTA SALAD

1 (12-ounce) package fusilli (use gluten-free pasta, if desired)

1 large zucchini, diced

⅓ cup diced English cucumber

1 pint cherry tomatoes, halved

¼ cup chopped fresh basil

⅓ cup fresh goat cheese (chèvre), crumbled (optional)

ZESTY HERB DRESSING

¼ cup extra-virgin olive oil

3 tablespoons distilled white vinegar

1 teaspoon honey or maple syrup

1½ teaspoons dried oregano

1 small shallot, finely chopped

1 teaspoon Dijon mustard (wine- and sulfite-free)

½ teaspoon kosher salt, or more to taste

¼ teaspoon crushed red pepper flakes

Freshly ground black pepper

To make the Summer Pasta Salad, bring a large pot of salted water to a boil. Add pasta and cook according to package directions. Drain and immediately run the pasta under cold water to keep it al dente. Drain again and transfer to a large bowl. Add the zucchini, cucumber, tomatoes, basil, and goat cheese (if using) and toss together.

To make the Zesty Herb Dressing, in a small bowl, whisk together the oil, vinegar, honey or maple syrup, oregano, shallot, mustard, salt, and red pepper flakes. Add about half of the dressing to the bowl with the pasta and vegetables and toss well.

Right before serving, add the remaining dressing, season to taste with more salt and black pepper, and toss again.

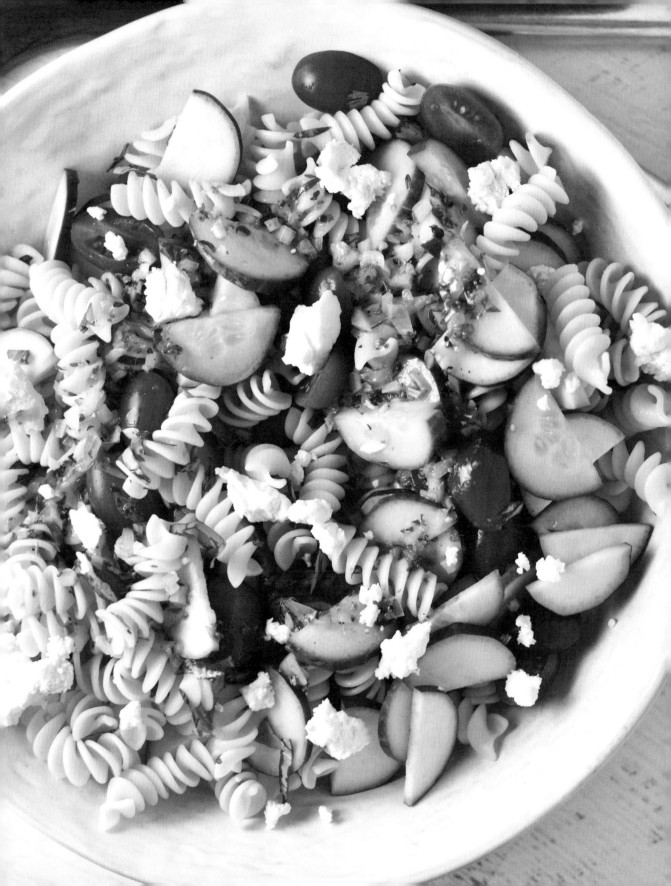

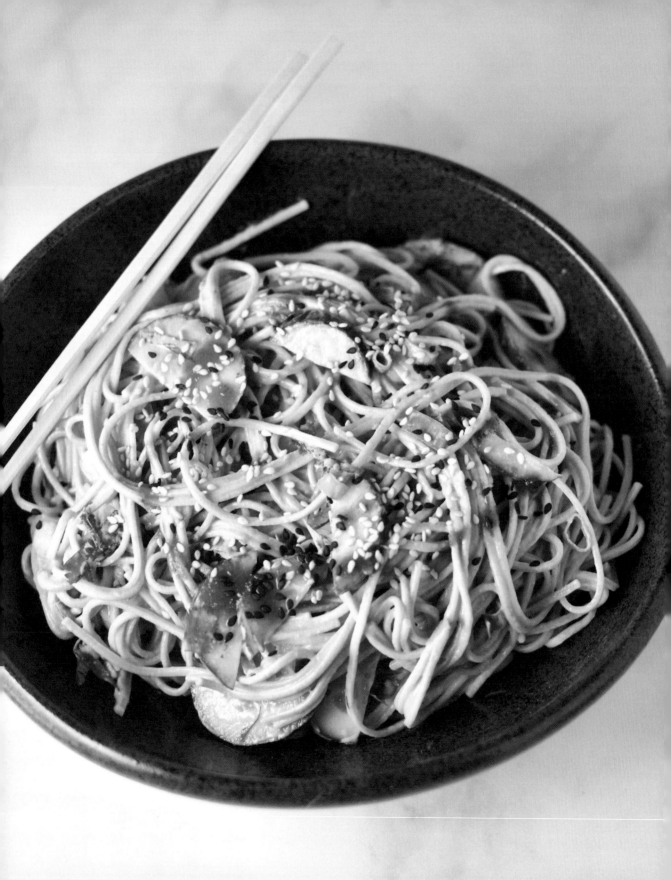

Chilled Soba Noodle Salad

MAKES 4 TO 6 SIDE-DISH OR 2 MAIN SERVINGS

Asian food became one of the things I missed the most on a migraine diet, but I've developed some recipes to help—like this one. Here, cold soba noodles are a wonderful substitute for peanut noodles on a hot summer day. Coconut aminos made from the sap of a coconut blossom is my favorite substitute for soy sauce. If you want to ensure you are eating gluten-free, make sure to buy 100 percent buckwheat noodles. (Some soba noodles are combined with wheat.) The taste of the sunflower seed butter can make or break this recipe, and brands really fluctuate in taste. Make sure you like the sunflower seed butter you're using before giving this recipe a try. I used Trader Joe's Sunflower Seed Spread which is unsweetened and lightly salted. Pretty Thai makes a clean sweet chili sauce. If you can't find a safe brand, you may need to add 1 or 2 teaspoons of honey to the sauce.

---

8 ounces buckwheat soba noodles or rice noodles

2 tablespoons toasted sesame oil, plus more as needed

2 tablespoons sesame seeds

2 tablespoons tahini

2 tablespoons unsweetened sunflower seed butter

2 tablespoons distilled white vinegar

2 teaspoons coconut aminos

1½ teaspoons ground ginger

1–2 tablespoons cold water

Honey (optional)

1 cup sliced English cucumber

½ cup chopped green onions

¼ cup chopped fresh cilantro

Sriracha (sulfite-, citrus-, and MSG-free), sweet chili sauce, and salt to taste

Cook the soba noodles according to package directions, drain well, and toss with a little bit of toasted sesame oil to prevent the noodles from sticking together.

Meanwhile, in a small dry skillet toast the sesame seeds over low heat until lightly browned, 2 to 3 minutes. Transfer to a plate and set aside to cool.

In a large bowl, mix together the 2 tablespoons sesame oil, tahini, sunflower seed butter, coconut aminos, vinegar, and ginger. Add 1 to 2 tablespoons or two of cold water to thin it out to a sauce consistency. Taste and add salt or honey, if desired. Add the noodles, cucumber, green onions, and cilantro. Toss well. Add salt to taste. Top with Sriracha and/or sweet chili sauce to taste. Sprinkle with the toasted sesame seeds and serve.

> **CONDIMENTS TIP** Some brands of coconut aminos are fermented, so if you're still in a chronic state, I would recommend just leaving it out until you feel you're ready to expand the diet a little more. Sriracha can be tough to find without sulfites. I can occasionally find a good brand in Whole Foods, but my favorites are Fix or Lingham's, both of which can be ordered from Amazon.

Pepita-Poppyseed Chicken Salad

MAKES 2 SERVINGS

This is my favorite lunch of all time! Perhaps it's a Southern thing, but I consider myself to be a chicken salad connoisseur. It always bums me out how many grocery stores and restaurants add nuts to theirs. This version with pepitas makes me wonder how no one else has caught on to this wonderful substitute. I prefer red grapes in this recipe, but some find them to be more of a trigger than green. This could potentially point to a tannin issue for you. But both are allowed on a migraine diet and can be enjoyed freely as long as you don't notice an increase in symptoms. Every once in a while, I like to switch them up for fresh pomegranate seeds.

¼ cup raw pepitas (pumpkin seeds)

¼ cup migraine-friendly mayonnaise

2 teaspoons distilled white vinegar

1½ teaspoons honey

½ teaspoon poppyseeds

¼ teaspoon kosher salt

2 cups shredded roasted chicken

1 celery stalk, diced

1 green onion, chopped

½ cup grapes, halved

Freshly ground black pepper to taste

To toast the pepitas, place them in a dry small skillet and cook over medium-low heat, stirring often, until lightly toasted, 3 to 4 minutes total. Transfer to a plate to cool.

In a large bowl, whisk together the mayonnaise, vinegar, honey, poppyseeds, and salt until blended. Add the chicken, celery, green onion, grapes, and toasted pepitas. Stir to combine. Season with pepper to taste. Refrigerate for 30 minutes for the best flavor, then serve.

> **NAKED ROTISSERIE CHICKEN** Many of the freshly cooked rotisserie chickens we see in the deli sections of grocery stores contain MSG, but I've found there are quite a few supermarkets that sell "naked chickens." Naked chickens mean they are either simply roasted or are only seasoned with salt and pepper. They're available at Whole Foods and Sprouts, or just double check the labels at the local grocery store.

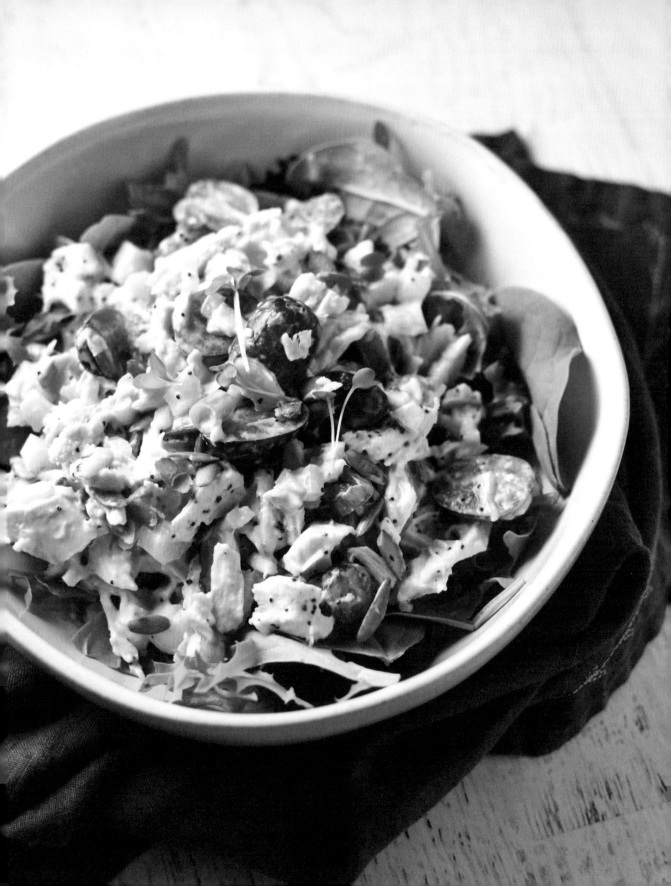

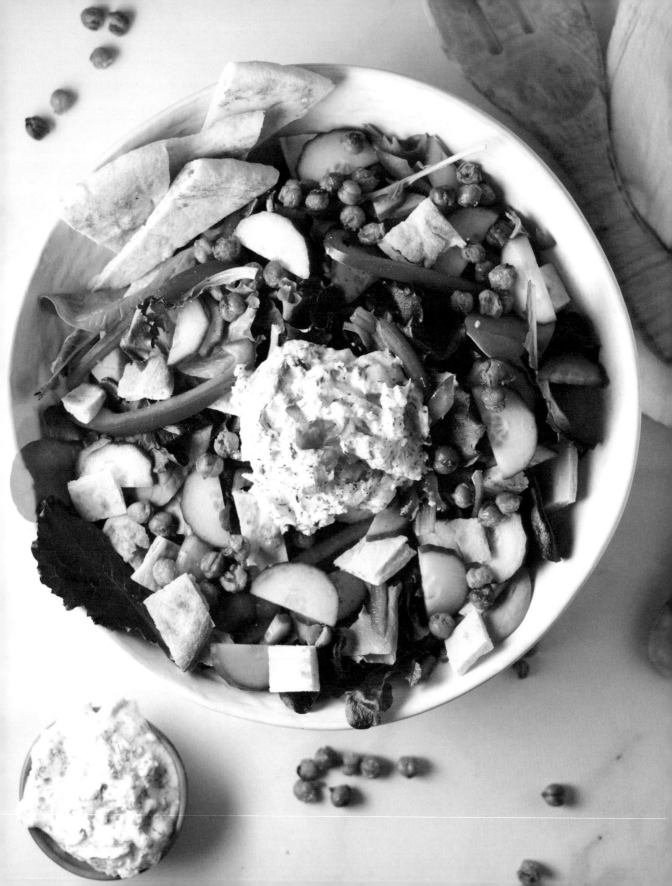

Mediterranean Pita Salad with Faux Tzatziki

MAKES 4 MAIN-DISH SERVINGS

Tzatziki—Greek-style garlic-yogurt-cucumber sauce or dip—was one of my favorite food items before I began this migraine-diet journey. Sadly, for me, yogurt ended up being a huge personal trigger. Even to this day, now that I've been able to add countless foods back, yogurt still makes my head feel slow and fuzzy when I eat it (though previously, it used to trigger a full-on vertigo attack). Luckily, I found a hack: blending cottage cheese gives you a nice, smooth texture that is similar to yogurt, and Daisy brand makes a cottage cheese without live cultures. If you haven't tried fried chickpeas yet… woah. These are addictive little guys that will be your new favorite snack.

FAUX TZATZIKI
¾ cup cottage cheese
  (without live cultures)
⅔ cup grated, unpeeled
  English cucumber
1 clove garlic, minced
1 tablespoon distilled white
  vinegar
1½ tablespoons fresh dill
  or 2 teaspoons dried dill

FRIED CHICKPEAS
Canola or grapeseed oil
1 (15-ounce) can chickpeas,
  drained and thoroughly dried
Kosher salt and freshly ground
  black pepper

PITA SALAD
1–2 pita or naan breads
  (made without yogurt)
1 (6-ounce) package mixed
  greens
1 red bell pepper, sliced
Chopped English cucumber
  (use the remaining cucumber
  from the Faux Tzatziki)

To make the Faux Tzatziki, place the cottage cheese in a food processor and blend until smooth, about 1 minute. Transfer to a serving bowl. Wrap the grated cucumber in a couple layers of paper towels or dish towels; squeeze out the excess moisture. Transfer to the bowl with the blended cottage cheese. Add garlic, vinegar, and dill; stir to combine. Cover and chill for at least 15 minutes.

To make the Fried Chickpeas, pour oil into a large skillet to a depth of ¼ inch. Heat over medium-high until it sizzles when you flick a bit of water into it. Add the dry chickpeas and fry, tossing occasionally with a slotted spoon, until browned on all sides, about 15 minutes total. Use the slotted spoon to transfer to paper towels to drain. Sprinkle with a little salt and pepper.

To make the Pita Salad, preheat the oven to 400°F and place the pita or naan bread directly on the center oven rack while the oven heats. Once the oven reaches 400°F, remove the bread and allow to cool. Chop into bite-size pieces.

In a large bowl, combine the mixed greens, red pepper, cucumber, pita pieces, and fried chickpeas; toss well. Divide the salad among serving plates, top each with a dollop of Faux Tzatziki, and serve.

Simple Tuna Salad

MAKES 2 SERVINGS

Easy to whip up for lunch or dinner, this tuna salad is simple yet satisfying. Serve on a bed of mixed greens, use radish slices or water crackers for dipping, or build a tuna sandwich. Let's be honest: my favorite way to serve this is with a ton of extra-crispy salted potato chips to balance out how healthy it is... but that's between you and me. If you can't find jicama, radishes can be substituted for a similar crunch.

---

1 (3-ounce) can tuna packed in water only

¼ cup peeled and chopped jicama

2 tablespoons chopped English cucumber

1 small green onion, chopped

2 tablespoons migraine-friendly mayonnaise

½ teaspoon chopped fresh dill or ¼ teaspoon dried dill

¼ teaspoon freshly ground black pepper

Kosher salt

Crackers (gluten-free, if desired) and sliced red radishes for serving

Drain the tuna and flake it into a small bowl. Add the jicama, cucumber, and green onion; stir to combine. Add the mayonnaise, dill, pepper, and salt to taste; stir until fully combined. Feel free to eat right away, but this is best when chilled for 30 minutes so the flavors have time to blend. Serve with crackers and radishes for dipping.

FRESH VS. CANNED There is some debate about canned tuna on a migraine diet, since it's not really "fresh." Obviously, it would be best to cook a fresh tuna yourself, but realistically that's not always an option. Tyramine is essentially derived from the natural bacteria present in food. As foods are exposed to warm temperatures or just plain oxygen over time, they can develop higher amounts of bacteria, leading to an increase in tyramine. With canned foods, however, there is no bacteria present in the food, protecting it until you open it. If you do find yourself sensitive to canned items, it could potentially be the lining in the can, or what it's packaged with. Many tuna brands are also packed in broths or seasonings that contain MSG. You'll want to make sure you purchase one that's been packed in water (or alone in a bag) without seasonings.

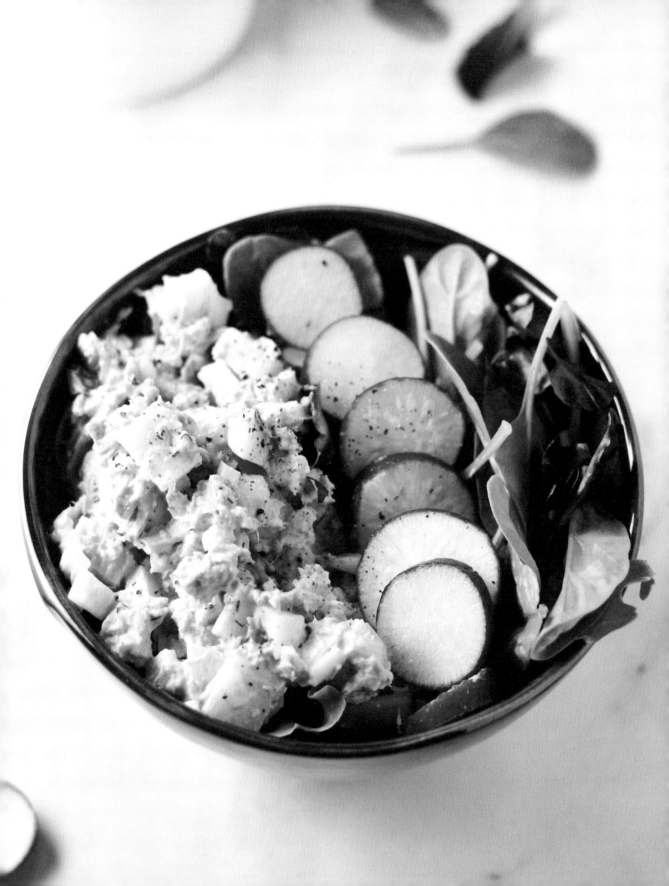

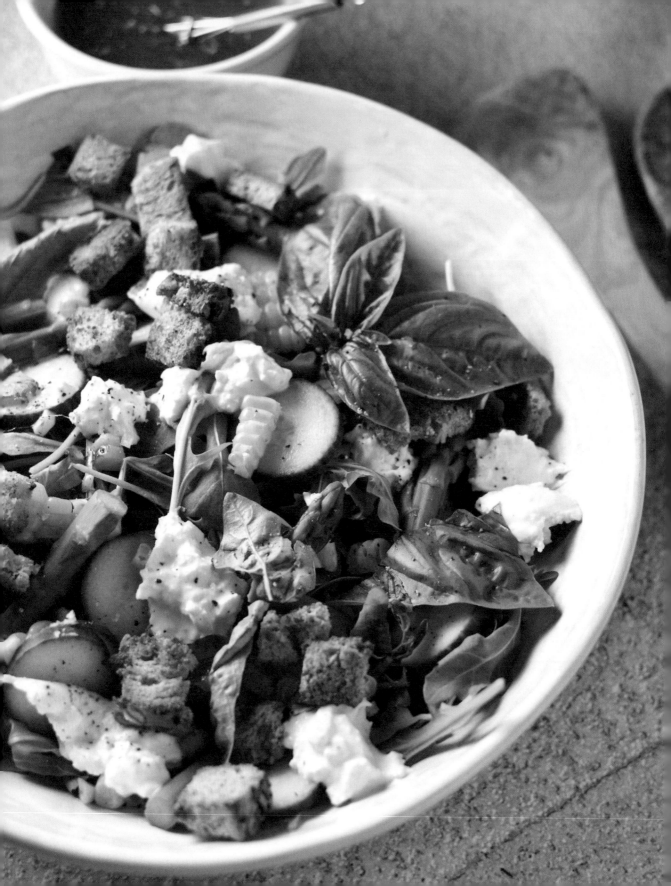

Burrata, Corn & Arugula Salad with Za'atar Croutons

MAKES 4 SIDE-DISH SERVINGS

I am obsessed with this salad. Its perfect combination of crunchy vegetables, super creamy burrata, and seasoned homemade croutons gives my heart a flutter! Didn't I tell you that you weren't going to feel deprived when cooking from this book? Za'atar is a Middle Eastern spice mixture made of sesame seeds, sumac, and thyme. You can typically find it in the bulk spice section of the grocery store or online. Most versions I've seen are migraine compliant, but be sure to always check your labels.

ZA'ATAR CROUTONS
2–3 slices migraine-safe bread
2–3 teaspoons olive oil
1½ teaspoons za'atar

OREGANO DRESSING
¼ cup plus 2 tablespoons extra-virgin olive oil
3 tablespoons distilled white vinegar
1 tablespoon apple juice
1 tablespoon minced shallot
2 teaspoons Dijon mustard (wine- and sulfite-free)
1½ teaspoons dried oregano
Kosher salt and freshly ground black pepper

SALAD
2 ears fresh corn, shucked
1 teaspoon olive oil
Kosher salt and freshly ground black pepper
6–8 asparagus spears
½ (5-ounce) package arugula
½ English cucumber, sliced
1 (4-ounce) ball burrata, drained and torn into pieces

To make the Za'atar Croutons, preheat the oven to 400°F. Cut the bread slices into 1-inch cubes and place in a bowl. Add the olive oil and za'atar and toss to coat evenly. Spread the bread cubes onto a baking sheet and bake until lightly browned, tossing occasionally, 7 to 10 minutes. Set aside.

To make the Oregano Dressing, in a small bowl, combine the olive oil, vinegar, apple juice, shallot, mustard, and oregano; whisk until smooth. Season to taste with salt and pepper.

To make the Burrata, Corn & Arugula Salad, position the oven rack in the top position and set the broiler to high. Place the corn ears on a baking sheet and rub with 1 teaspoon olive oil. Sprinkle with kosher salt and pepper to taste. Broil the corn, turning it every 5 to 6 minutes, until there's a nice char on both sides, 10 to 12 minutes total. Remove from the oven and allow to cool. Remove the kernels and transfer to a large bowl.

Meanwhile, bring a small pot of salted water to a boil and prepare an ice bath. Cut the asparagus spears into 1-inch pieces. Add the asparagus pieces to the boiling water and cook for 1½ minutes. Using a slotted spoon, immediately remove the asparagus and place in the ice bath to stop the cooking. Drain the asparagus pieces and pat them dry. Add to the bowl with the corn. Add the arugula, cucumber and burrata pieces. Add Oregano Dressing to taste (there may be a little left over) and toss well. Top with the Za'atar Croutons and serve right away.

Curried Carrot & Sweet Potato Soup

MAKES 4 TO 6 SERVINGS

This is a perfect soup for using up those lonely carrots and sweet potatoes you have left over from the week. Most of these items are pantry staples, and this recipe requires very little effort. It's warm, somewhat spicy, slightly sweet, and very comforting.

---

1 tablespoon olive oil

1 pound carrots, peeled and chopped

2 cups peeled and chopped sweet potatoes (about 1 medium-sized potato)

2 shallots, roughly chopped

3 cloves garlic, roughly chopped

2 teaspoons kosher salt, plus more to taste

1½ tablespoons curry powder

¼ teaspoon ground ginger

4 cups Chicken Stock (page 81) or Vegetable Broth (page 80)

1 tablespoon sunflower seed butter

Freshly ground black pepper to taste

Microgreens for garnish (optional)

In a large pot, warm the olive oil over medium heat. Add the carrots, sweet potatoes, shallots, garlic, and salt, and cook, stirring often, until the vegetables are slightly browned, about 10 minutes. Stir in the curry powder and ginger. Pour in the stock or broth and bring to a simmer. Simmer until all the vegetables have softened, about 20 minutes. Carefully pour the soup into a blender, or use an immersion blender, and blend until smooth. Return the soup to the original pot, place over low heat, and stir in the sunflower seed butter. Warm until smooth and heated through. Season to taste.

Ladle the soup into bowls. Garnish with microgreens, if desired, and freshly ground pepper, and serve hot.

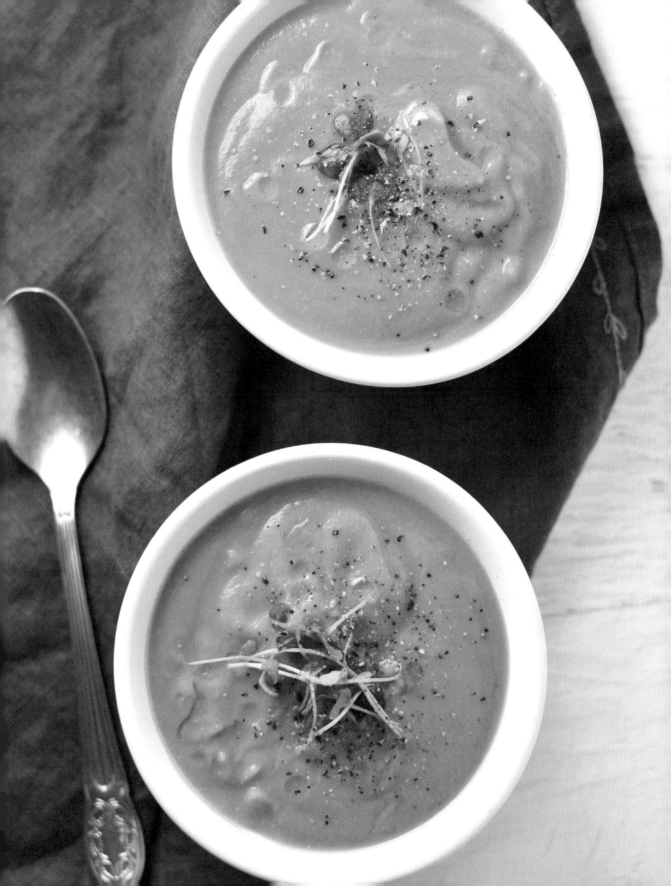

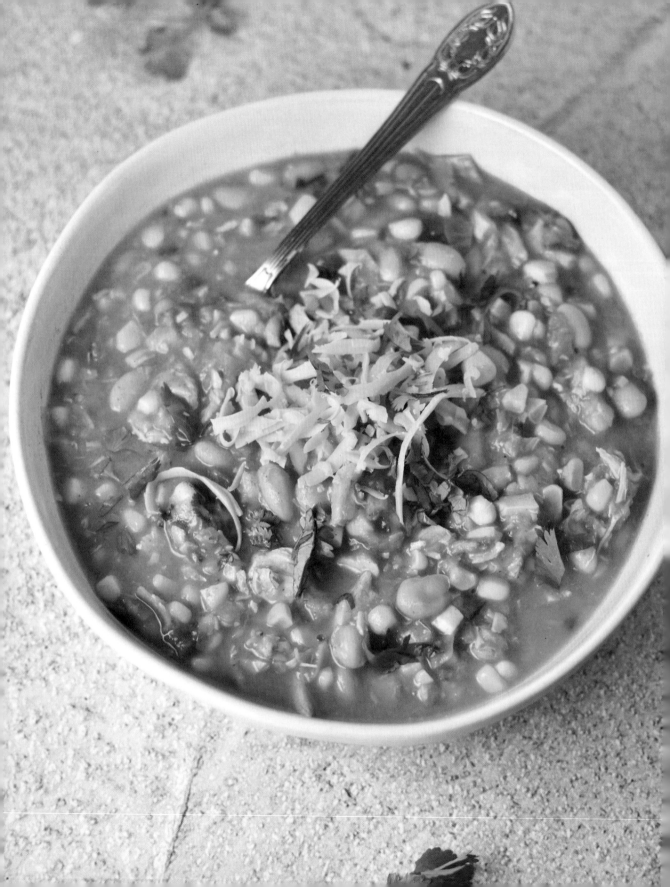

White Bean Chicken Chili

MAKES 4 TO 6 SERVINGS

The perfect option for winter weather, this tomato-less chili uses Great Northern beans, which are one of the varieties of beans allowed on a migraine diet. Blending one can of the beans provides some creaminess without any dairy. This one is a go-to for meal prepping—you can make it up to 1 month ahead of time, freeze it in individual bags, and have it ready for lunch or dinner during the week. Leeks can be quite sandy in between the layers, so you want to make sure you clean them well. Trim away the ends, where the light green turns darker, and the bottoms near the "hair." Then slice them in half lengthwise and separate all the little pieces. Place them in a bowl of cool water and allow the sediment to fall to the bottom, then rinse one final time.

---

2 (15.5-ounce) cans Great Northern beans, drained

4 cups Chicken Stock (page 81) or Vegetable Broth (page 80)

1 tablespoon olive oil

2 leeks (white and pale-green parts only), chopped

1 poblano chile, seeds and ribs removed, minced

1 jalapeño chile, seeds and ribs removed, minced

2 cloves garlic, minced

1 cup frozen or fresh corn kernels

2 teaspoons ground cumin

1½ teaspoons smoked paprika

1 teaspoon chili powder

1 teaspoon kosher salt

1 "naked" rotisserie chicken or 3 cooked chicken breasts, meat removed from the bone and chopped (4 cups total)

Fresh chopped cilantro and shredded American cheese (optional) for garnish

In a blender or food processor, combine half of the beans with 1 cup of the stock or broth. In batches, if necessary, blend until smooth and creamy, then set aside.

In a large pot, warm the olive oil over medium heat. Add the leeks and sauté until softened, 3 to 4 minutes. Add the poblano, jalapeño, garlic, and corn; sauté another 5 minutes. Add the cumin, smoked paprika, chili powder, salt, and remaining whole beans. Stir to combine. Add the chopped chicken, remaining 3 cups of stock or broth, and the blended bean mixture. Simmer over low heat for 30 minutes to develop the flavors.

Ladle the chili into bowls and garnish with cilantro and cheese, if desired. Serve hot.

Creamy Cauliflower & Leek Soup

MAKES 4 TO 5 SERVINGS

This soup is my knockoff version of potato leek, but it won't make you feel so heavy after eating it. What makes this soup special is the blended cauliflower, which allows this soup to be creamy without adding a ton of dairy. The butter gives this recipe just enough richness to feel a little decadent. Roasting the cauliflower is essential to bringing its that nutty, delicious flavor. I love to add pepitas for a bit of crunch, but toasted bread or croutons would also be wonderful with this soup.

---

2 pounds fresh cauliflower florets

3 tablespoons olive oil, divided

2 teaspoons kosher salt, plus more to taste, divided

Freshly ground black pepper

1½ cups chopped leeks (white and pale-green parts only)

3 cloves garlic, chopped

2 tablespoons unsalted butter

4 cups Vegetable Broth (page 80) or Chicken Stock (page 81)

2 teaspoons distilled white vinegar

1 tablespoon chopped fresh parsley, plus more for garnish

1 teaspoon dried thyme

Pepitas (pumpkin seeds), toasted, for garnish

Preheat the oven to 425°F. On a large baking sheet, toss the cauliflower florets with 2 tablespoons olive oil, 1 teaspoon kosher salt, and pepper to taste. Roast until lightly browned, tossing halfway through, about 30 minutes.

In a large pot, warm the remaining 1 tablespoon olive oil over medium heat. Add the leeks, garlic, and remaining 1 teaspoon kosher salt. Cook until leeks have softened and are somewhat translucent, stirring often, 2 to 3 minutes. Transfer the cooked leeks and garlic to a blender along with the butter, broth or stock, and roasted cauliflower. Blend until smooth (an immersion blender also works).

Return the mixture to the pot and bring to a low simmer. Add the vinegar, parsley, and thyme. Season to taste with salt and pepper. Ladle the soup into bowls and garnish with toasted pepitas and chopped parsley. Serve hot.

> **HIDDEN MSG** Making your own soup may seem like a hassle, but it really is so much better for your head health than eating canned or processed soups. If you've ever looked at the ingredient labels on prepared soups, even on the best soups at high-end markets, there always seem to be hidden triggers lurking along with secretive names for MSG. This is often because places just don't take the time to make their own stocks and broths. Take it from me: it's very empowering to know exactly what's in the food you're eating and creating.

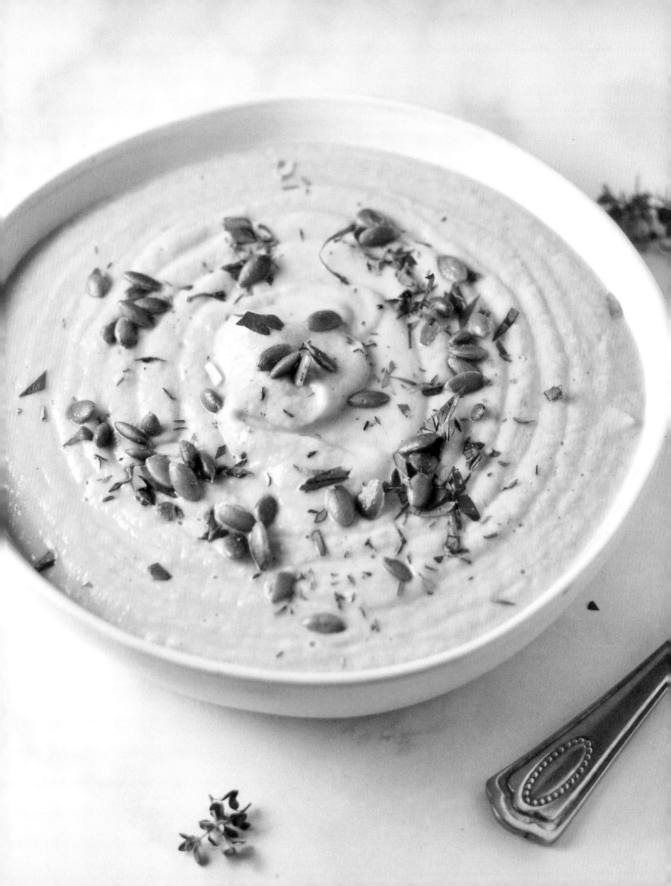

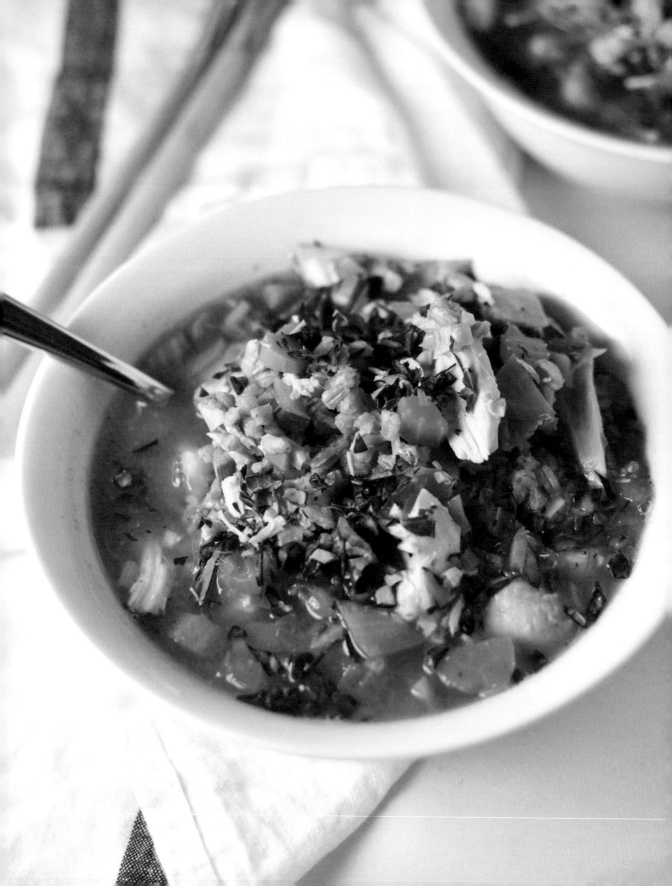

Farro & Lemongrass Chicken Soup

MAKES ABOUT 6 SERVINGS

Hearty, healthy, and delicious, this is the adult version of chicken noodle soup. Farro isn't gluten free, so if you'd like to adapt this recipe, you could either leave it out or add GF noodles later in the cooking process. This soup would be fabulous in vegetarian form as well, so you could also simply leave out the chicken. Lemongrass can be found in most grocery stores, either fresh or in a tube. It adds a lovely lemony flavor without the addition of citrus, which is off limits on a migraine diet. If you like, use meat picked from a "naked" rotisserie chicken.

1 tablespoon olive oil

1 cup chopped celery (about 2 stalks)

1 cup chopped leeks (about 2 stalks; white and pale-green parts only)

1 cup chopped carrots (about 1 large carrot)

4 cloves garlic, minced

2 lemongrass stalks, ends trimmed to about 4-inch pieces, halved lengthwise

2 teaspoons kosher salt, plus more to taste

1 teaspoon freshly ground black pepper, plus more to taste

7–8 cups Chicken Stock (page 81) or Vegetable Broth (page 80), plus more if needed to thin the soup

½ cup pearled farro

1 teaspoon dried thyme

½ teaspoon ground sage

2–3 cups chopped cooked chicken

1–2 cups roughly chopped kale (save a few pieces for garnish)

In a large pot, warm the olive oil over medium heat. Add the celery, leeks, and carrots and sauté until vegetables have softened and lightly browned, 8 to 10 minutes. Add the garlic, lemongrass stalks, salt, and pepper. Sauté for another 2 minutes. Add the stock or broth, farro, thyme, and sage. Bring to a boil. Reduce the heat to medium-low and simmer until farro is tender, about 30 minutes.

Remove the lemongrass stalks and stir in the chicken and kale. Simmer until the kale is softened and slightly wilted, another 5 minutes. Farro continues to soak up liquid, so thin the soup with additional stock or broth if needed. Add additional salt and pepper to taste.

Ladle the soup into bowls and garnish with extra kale. Serve hot.

Fish Chowder

MAKES 4 TO 6 SERVINGS

I'm a firm believer that adding cream to just about anything makes it instantly delicious. It's true with this recipe, which is one of my all-time favorite soups. Pretty much anything labeled "chowder" is like comfort in a bowl. A firm fish, like cod or haddock, works best here so it doesn't fall apart.

---

1 tablespoon olive oil

2 cups diced unpeeled Yukon Gold potatoes (about ½-inch cubes)

1 cup chopped leeks (about 2 stalks; white and pale-green parts only)

½ cup chopped carrot (about ½ carrot)

½ cup chopped celery (about 1 stalk)

1 cup fresh or frozen corn kernels

2 teaspoons kosher salt

1 teaspoon freshly ground black pepper

4 cups Vegetable Broth (page 80)

1 pound cod or haddock, deboned and skin removed, cut into 1-inch chunks

2 teaspoons dried thyme

2 bay leaves

1 teaspoon paprika

1 teaspoon dry mustard

½ cup heavy cream (carrageenan-free)

In a large pot, warm the oil over medium-high heat. Add the diced potatoes and sauté until they are lightly browned and starting to soften, about 5 minutes. Add the leeks, carrots, celery, corn, salt, and pepper. Sauté until the leeks are translucent and the other vegetables are fragrant and softened, another 5 to 7 minutes. Add the broth and bring to a simmer. Add the fish, thyme, bay leaves, paprika, and mustard and simmer on low heat until the fish is fully cooked through, about 15 minutes.

Stir in the cream and simmer for another 5 minutes. Ladle the chowder into bowls and serve hot.

> **HIDDEN INGREDIENTS** Carrageenan, which is derived from red seaweed, is on the avoid list because seaweed is high in glutamate. Often used as a thickener in milk or cream, carrageenan can be a trigger in individuals who are sensitive to MSG.

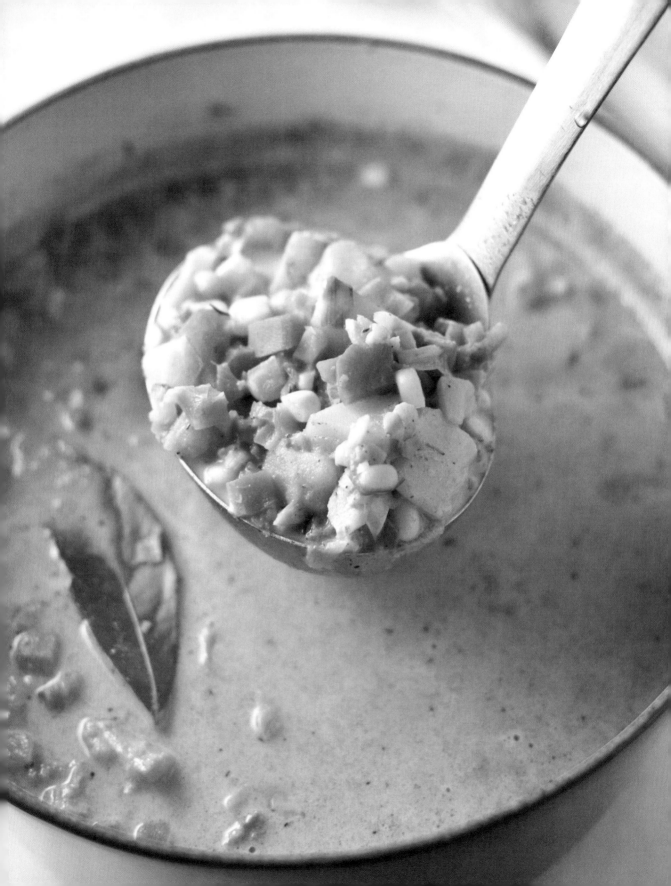

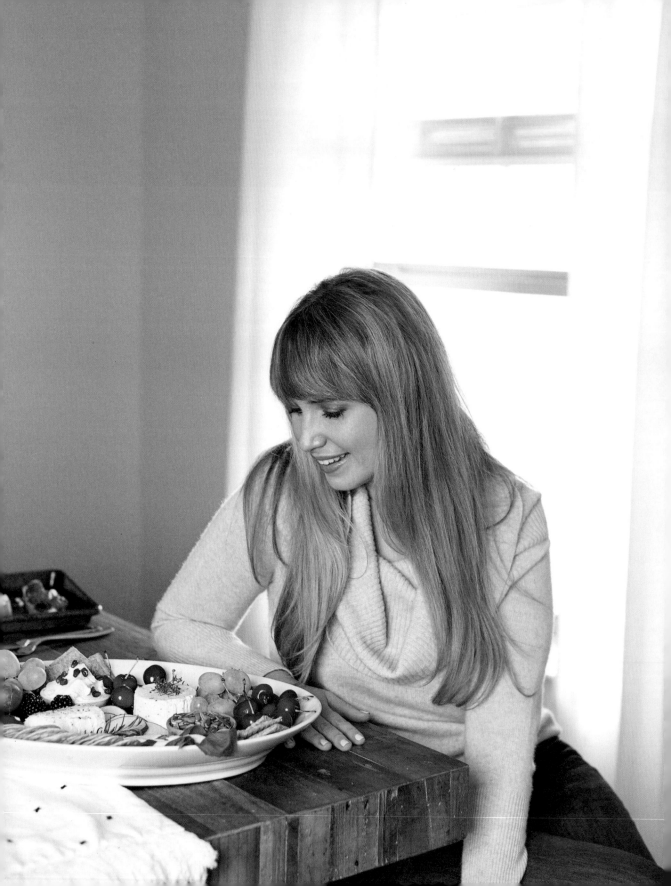

Snacks & Starters

I love a good party, but I quickly found out that migraine diets and other people's parties don't mix very well. I have no idea what's in anyone else's food, and the community table can quickly become a minefield. This is why it's always good to: (1) bring at least one migraine-safe dish you can eat or (2) have the party at your place.

I realize hosting a party sounds exhausting, but hear me out. You get to control the lighting situation and what time everyone arrives and leaves. You don't even have to worry about any rogue tropical-scented candles. The food doesn't need to be complicated either. Several of my ideas involve minimal hands-on time—like the Queso Dip, Crispy Taco-Spiced Wings, and the MSG-Free Party Mix. The Migraine-Safe Cheese Board is all about arranging store-bought items into a beautiful platter that will wow any guest (and they won't even miss aged cheese).

If the only party you want to have is with yourself, give the Spinach Artichoke Flatbreads a try for dinner one night. I keep migraine-safe pita or naan bread in my freezer, so such recipes are ready to whip up at a moment's notice for an easy weeknight dinner.

The Seed Butter Energy Balls and Pepita Protein Bars are also two of my freezer staples, and I just pop them out when I need a quick breakfast or snack on the go.

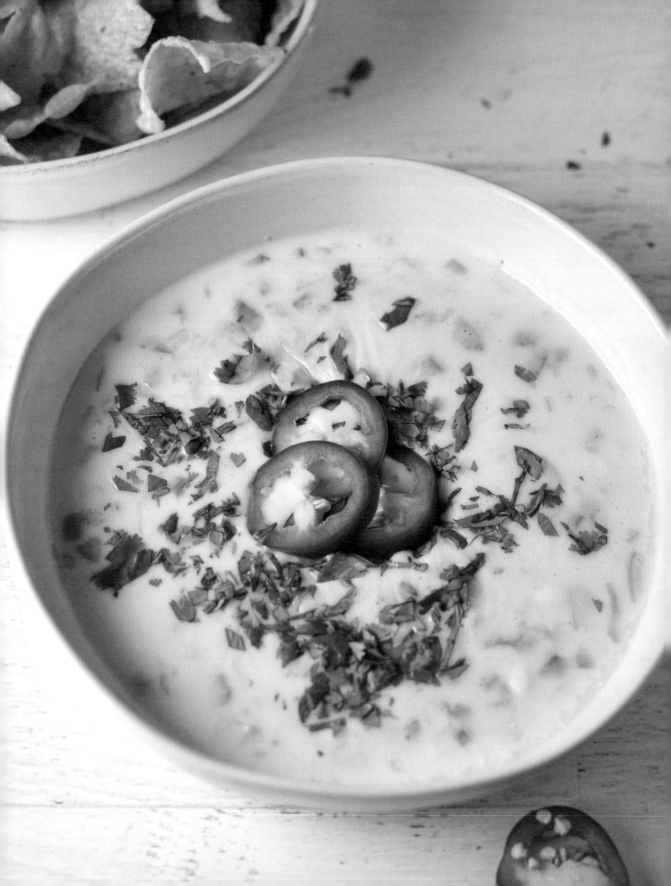

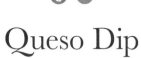

Queso Dip

MAKES 4 SERVINGS

Living with migraine and being on an elimination diet can feel very isolating at times. I used to often turn down dinner with friends because I couldn't control what I was going to eat and only had a select few restaurants I really trusted. That's when I started having more people over to my house. I could control the food, lighting, and scents. While it does seem like a lot of work, you don't always have to have a full menu. Simple snacks like these can be a crowd pleaser without a ton of work. In Texas, queso—melted cheese dip—is a way of life. And nothing beats real, homemade queso. After trying this recipe, you'll never want Velveeta again.

½ cup whole milk

½ pound good-quality white American cheese, shredded

½ shallot, finely chopped

¼ cup chopped fresh cilantro, plus more for garnish

½ teaspoon kosher salt

¼ teaspoon ground cumin

1 jalapeño chile, seeds and ribs removed, finely chopped (optional; set aside 2–3 thin slices of jalapeño for garnish)

Corn tortilla chips for serving

In a medium saucepan, warm the milk over medium heat. Once the milk is warm, add the cheese a small handful at a time, whisking thoroughly until smooth. If you add it all at once, the cheese might clump together.

When all the cheese has melted, add the shallot, cilantro, salt, cumin, and chopped jalapeño (if using).

When you're ready to serve, pour the queso into a heatproof serving bowl and garnish with additional cilantro and jalapeño slices (if using). Serve warm with tortilla chips. The cheese will harden as it cools, so microwave the dip in 30-second increments to remelt, stirring often.

> **HEAD-FRIENDLY DIPPERS** There are so many options for dippers that are both migraine safe and gluten free. Traditional corn tortilla chips (without seasonings) or blue corn chips work really well for this recipe. If you'd like to use vegetables, jicama or radishes would provide an enticing crunch and neutral flavor. Warmed corn or flour tortillas are also fantastic.

Pepita Protein Bars

MAKES 12 BARS

This recipe saved me many times when I first started the HYH diet or while traveling. I recommend making a big batch of these, packaging them individually, and storing them in the freezer so you can reach for them as a quick snack. Having migraine-safe snacks on hand will keep you from automatically going for something that may be a trigger food just because you're tired and hungry. I also love these for a quick breakfast on the run. They will soften the longer you leave them out at room temperature, so keep that in mind.

1½ cups quick-cooking oats (certified gluten-free, if desired)

1 cup raw pepitas (pumpkin seeds)

¼ cup raw hemp seeds

½ cup honey

¾ cup sunflower seed butter

1½ teaspoons ground cinnamon

¼ teaspoon ground nutmeg

2 teaspoons vanilla extract

Preheat the oven to 300°F. Line an 8-by-8-inch baking pan with a parchment paper overhang and set aside. Spread the oats on a baking sheet and toast in the oven for 15 minutes. Remove the oats from the oven and toss them around on the baking sheet, then add the pepitas and hemp seeds. Toast for another 10 to 15 minutes, checking often to make sure the seeds don't burn. Remove from the oven and let cool.

In a small saucepan, warm the honey over medium-low heat until it thins outs and starts to simmer, about 3 minutes. Remove from heat and add the sunflower seed butter, stirring until combined. Transfer the mixture to a large bowl and add the cinnamon, nutmeg, vanilla, and toasted oat-seed mixture. Spread the mixture evenly inside the prepared baking pan, pressing down firmly on top to make sure it reaches the edges. Place the pan in the refrigerator for 1 hour to firm.

Grasp the sides of the parchment and lift the bars out of the pan onto a cutting board. Using a sharp knife, cut them into 12 squares.

To store, I like to wrap these individually in wax paper or plastic wrap so I can grab one and go. You can store them for 1 to 2 months in the freezer (in a freezer-safe bag or container). If you're pulling from the freezer, allow them to sit at room temperature for a few minutes and they will soften enough to eat.

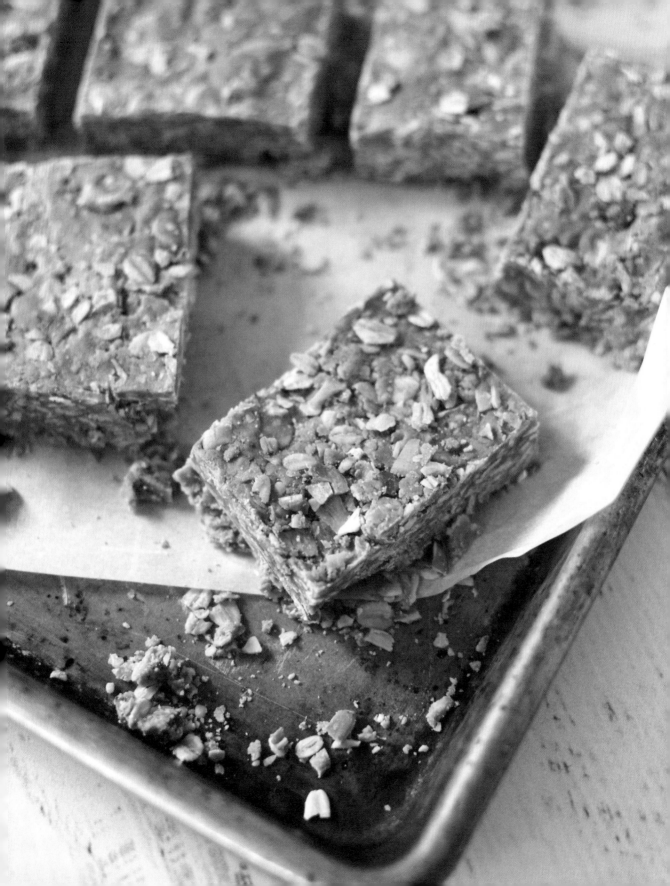

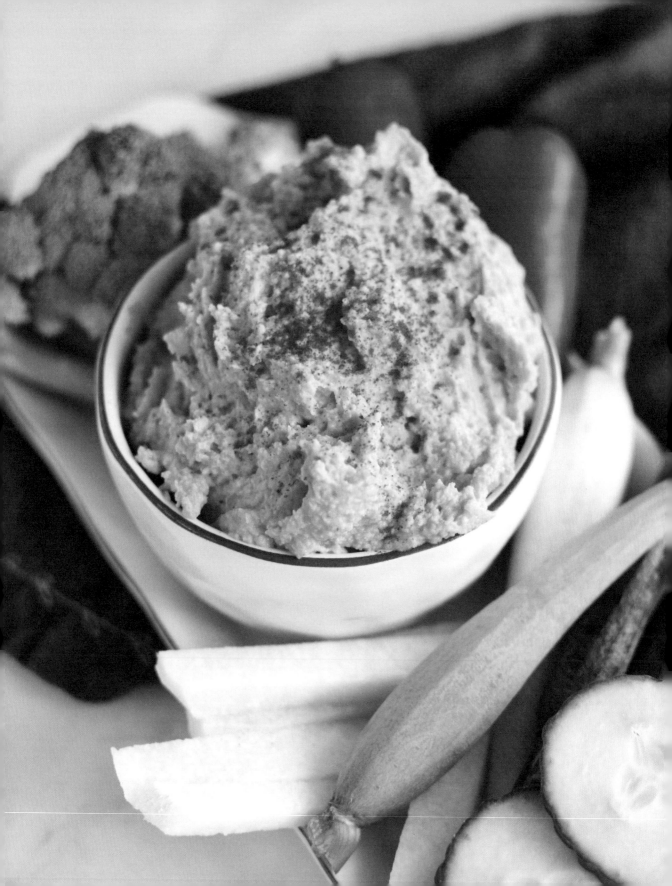

Smoky Carrot Hummus

MAKES 2 CUPS

If you're lucky, you can find safe hummus at the grocery store, but it's not always easy—many have lemon juice or additives. I love to use white vinegar and sumac to bump up the "citrus" flavor I'm missing whenever I make my own at home. A trick for super creamy hummus is to boil canned chickpeas for about 20 minutes with ½ teaspoon of baking soda. This softens the chickpeas and their skins, so the hummus has an incredibly smooth texture. I used to be one of those crazy people who popped each chickpea out of their skin, but the boiling essentially does the same thing, more easily. It's simple to figure out how to make good, traditional hummus with the tips above, so I wanted to give you something unique with this recipe. The carrot adds a hint of sweetness and pairs beautifully with the smoked paprika. If you love Southwestern flavors, you'll really enjoy this one.

---

1 (15-ounce) can chickpeas (garbanzo beans)

½ teaspoon baking soda

1 cup roughly chopped carrots (about 1 large carrot)

1 clove garlic

¼ cup distilled white vinegar

⅓ cup tahini

2–4 tablespoons ice water

1 teaspoon ground cumin

1 teaspoon smoked paprika

⅛ teaspoon chipotle chile powder

½ teaspoon kosher salt

2 tablespoons olive oil

Pita chips, celery sticks, radishes, cherry tomatoes, sliced cucumbers, and/or baby carrots for dipping

Drain the chickpeas and transfer to a small saucepan. Add just enough water to cover the chickpeas and add the baking soda. Bring to a boil over high heat, then reduce the heat to low, cover, and allow chickpeas to simmer until they look a little larger and are soft, with some skins falling off, about 20 minutes. Drain and let cool.

Meanwhile, add the carrots to another small saucepan, cover with water, and boil until softened, about 10 minutes. Drain into the same colander as the chickpeas and let cool.

In a food processor, combine the garlic and vinegar. Blend until the garlic is minced. Add the tahini and mix until smooth, then add ice water to thin the mixture out until smooth and creamy. Add the cumin, smoked paprika, chile powder, salt, and the softened chickpeas and carrots. Process everything until smooth and creamy. Transfer the hummus to a serving bowl, cover, and chill for roughly 30 minutes to allow the flavors to combine.

Serve with pita chips, celery, radishes, tomatoes, cucumbers… and even more carrots.

Bruschetta Board

MAKES 4 TO 6 APPETIZER SERVINGS PER LARGE BAGUETTE

Serve this at a party, and even non-sufferers will be wowed by your skills. Bruschetta has this magical way of saying, "I'm fancy!" without all the time and effort. Below are three ideas for migraine-friendly bruschetta appetizers, but the possibilities aren't just limited to these options. Use your imagination! The untopped crostini also freeze and reheat well if you just want a few pieces with a meal.

---

1 day-old baguette or other head-friendly, sturdy bread,
Olive oil

GRAPE, GOAT CHEESE & THYME

2 cups sliced red grapes
1 tablespoon olive oil
1 teaspoon fresh thyme leaves
Kosher salt and freshly ground black pepper
1 (4-ounce) package fresh goat cheese (chèvre)
Chopped fresh thyme

RED PEPPER & GOAT CHEESE

2 tablespoons olive oil
1 (16-ounce) jar roasted red peppers
1 (4-ounce) package fresh goat cheese (chèvre)
¼ cup thinly sliced fresh basil
Freshly ground black pepper and flaky sea salt to taste

PEACH, RICOTTA & BASIL

1 (15-ounce) package fresh ricotta cheese
1 peach, thinly sliced
¼ cup thinly sliced fresh basil
Freshly ground black pepper
Honey

To make the crostini, slice the bread at an angle. Position the oven rack 6 inches from broiler and preheat the broiler. Brush each bread slice on both sides with olive oil, arrange in a single layer on a baking sheet, and broil until lightly browned on each side, flipping halfway, 5 to 7 minutes total. Watch carefully to make sure they don't burn. Let cool.

To make the Grape, Goat Cheese & Thyme Bruschetta, preheat the oven to 425°F. On a baking sheet, toss the grapes with the olive oil, fresh thyme leaves, and a sprinkle of salt and pepper. Roast until the grapes have softened, about 20 minutes, and let cool slightly. Spread the goat cheese onto the crostini, then top with the roasted grapes. Garnish with fresh thyme leaves.

To make the Red Pepper & Goat Cheese Bruschetta, slice the peppers into ¼-inch-wide strips. Spread the crostini with goat cheese, top with red pepper strips, and garnish with basil, freshly ground black pepper, and sea salt.

To make the Peach, Ricotta & Basil Bruschetta, spread a layer of ricotta on each crostini. Place a peach slice on top of each crostini, then top with basil leaves, fresh black pepper, and a drizzle of honey.

> **BREAD ALTERNATIVES** If you cannot locate clean bread, consider using water crackers or thinly sliced large radishes, like watermelon radishes, for the "crostini."

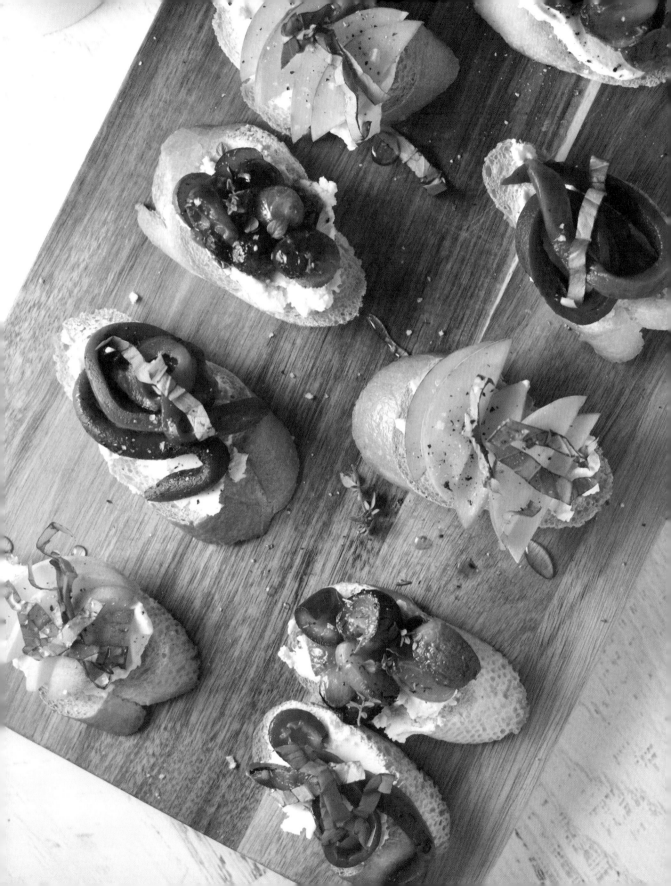

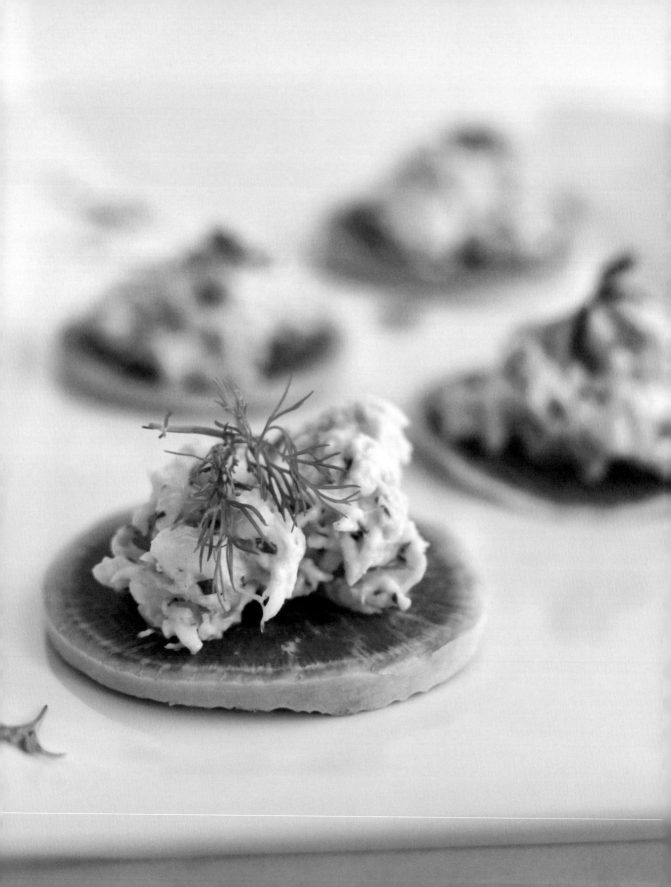

Crab Salad Bites

MAKES ABOUT 10 BITES

This best thing about the migraine diet (yes, there is a good part!) is that you can get a little adventurous with your eating. Once you start going to the grocery store and looking at all the things you can have, it really opens up possibilities. Watermelon radish was one of my discoveries. Whiteish green on the outside, it's very unassuming until you cut into it and the center is a stunning lime green with a hot pink center. Delicate in flavor, it makes a choice "toast" for those who are gluten free and who struggle to find a safe packaged cracker option. If you can't find watermelon radish, a red radish will do, but they will be bite-sized. Or you could serve this on a plain water cracker. For those who aren't a big fan of crab, use chopped, cooked shrimp for an easy substitute. If you would rather use dried spices, just halve the amount listed.

---

8 ounces fresh lump crabmeat, picked free of shells

¼ cup finely chopped celery (about 1 stalk)

1 tablespoon finely chopped shallot

2 teaspoons finely chopped fresh dill, plus more for garnish

1½ teaspoons finely chopped fresh parsley

1½ teaspoons finely chopped fresh chives

2 tablespoons migraine-friendly mayonnaise

1½ teaspoons Dijon mustard (wine- and sulfite-free)

Kosher salt and freshly ground black pepper

1–2 large radishes (such as watermelon radishes)

In a small bowl, combine the crabmeat, celery, shallot, dill, parsley, chives, mayonnaise, and mustard; mix well. Season to taste with salt and pepper. Cover and chill for 30 minutes to blend the flavors.

Cut the watermelon radish into ¼-inch-thick slices and arrange on a platter. Top each radish slice with chilled crab salad. Garnish with a little extra dill and serve.

Spinach Artichoke Flatbreads

MAKES 2 FLATBREADS

This "wait 24 hours to consume fresh bread" rule really throws a wrench in pizza night. The best way around this is to find a safe flatbread, like pita or naan. You have to be a little careful with naan bread because a lot of brands include yogurt, but I never have an issue with finding at least one safe option. If you're gluten free, Trader Joe's makes a delicious cauliflower crust that's small in diameter. As for cream cheese, you'll want to watch for additives like carrageenan. I recommend Arla or Organic Valley, but some store-name brands are also fine. Since my best friend is a vegetarian, I made this for my friends one girls' night and they couldn't get enough.

---

2 pita or naan breads (made without yogurt), purchased (thawed if frozen)

5 plain artichoke hearts, drained and rinsed well or thawed (if using jarred or canned, look for them in water only, no spices)

1 (10-ounce) bag fresh baby spinach

2 teaspoons olive oil

1 clove garlic, minced

3 ounces plain cream cheese (carrageenan-free)

½ teaspoon fresh black pepper

¼ teaspoon kosher salt

Chopped fresh basil for garnish

Crushed red pepper flakes for garnish (optional)

Preheat the oven to 425°F. Place the naan or pita directly on the middle oven rack and toast for 5 minutes until slightly crispy.

Meanwhile, roughly chop the artichoke hearts and spinach. In a large skillet, warm the olive oil over medium heat and add the garlic. Sauté until fragrant, about 1 minute. Add the artichoke hearts and spinach and cook, stirring, until the spinach is wilted, 2 to 3 minutes. Add the cream cheese, pepper, and salt. Stir until well blended.

Remove the flatbreads from the oven and place on a work surface. Spread the spinach-artichoke mixture on top of the toasted breads, dividing evenly. Place the flatbreads back into the oven, directly on the rack, and bake until browned and bubbly, another 5 to 7 minutes. If the flatbreads aren't brown enough on top for you, broil under high heat on the upper rack for 1 minute. Slice into appetizer-sized pieces, garnish with fresh basil and set out red pepper flakes for sprinkling, and serve.

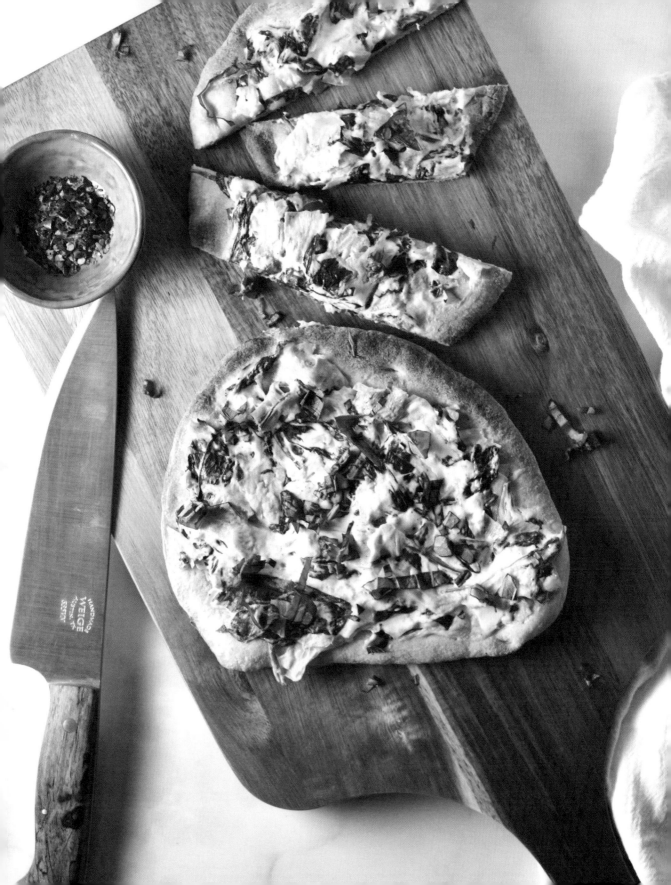

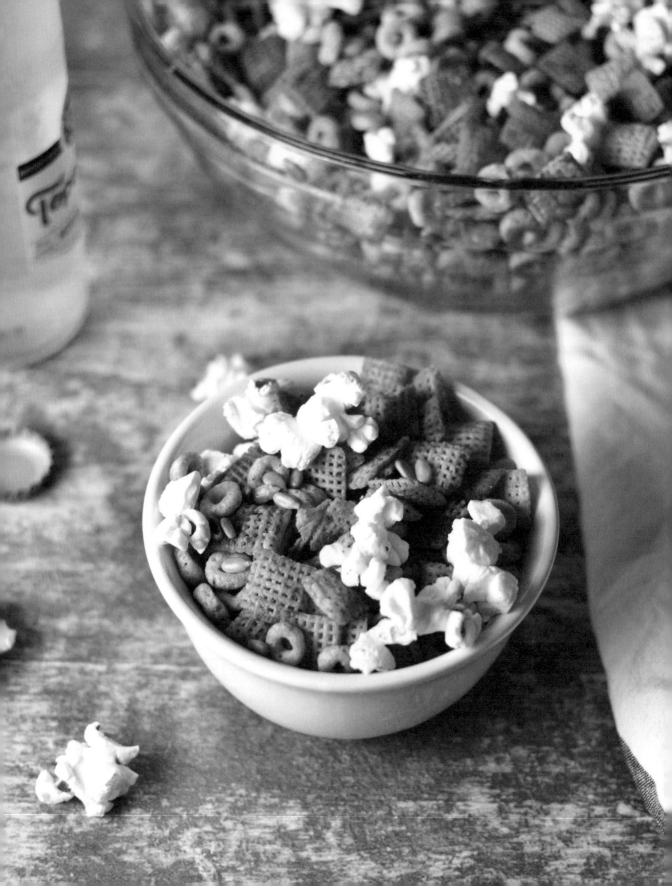

MSG-Free Party Mix

MAKES ABOUT 8 CUPS

One of my favorite website readers requested a Chex Mix recipe a while ago, saying it was the snack she missed the most after being diagnosed with migraine. (Finding this mix without MSG or soy sauce is impossible!) I wasn't quite sure how this one would turn out, but I was pleasantly surprised with the results. Coconut aminos isn't actually made from coconut, but from the sap of a coconut blossom. Many find they can tolerate this ingredient quite well as an alternative to soy sauce. If you don't have access to coconut aminos, just substitute homemade stock or broth.

4 cups plain Chex cereal (I use the rice and corn varieties)

1 cup unsalted sunflower seeds, toasted

5 tablespoons unsalted butter, melted

2 tablespoons coconut aminos or broth

1 tablespoon distilled white vinegar

2 teaspoons garlic powder

1 teaspoon celery seeds

1 teaspoon smoked paprika

1 teaspoon kosher salt

½ teaspoon chili powder

¼ teaspoon ground turmeric

3 cups plain Cheerios

1–2 cups plain popped popcorn

In a large microwave-safe bowl, combine the Chex, sunflower seeds, melted butter, coconut aminos, vinegar, garlic powder, celery seeds, smoked paprika, salt, chili powder, and turmeric. Microwave on high power for 2 minutes. Add the Cheerios to the bowl, then stir everything thoroughly. Microwave for another 2 minutes, then stir everything together again. Stir in the popcorn and microwave for 1 final minute.

Allow the party mix to cool before serving. It will be super crunchy at the point it is cool.

Migraine-Safe Cheese Board

MAKES ENOUGH FOR A CROWD OF GRATEFUL PEOPLE

I won't lie, I did miss aged cheese for a long time. I like to consider myself a cheese connoisseur—cheese is one of my favorite things in the world. (On our trip to Burgundy, servers would bring out cheese plates so large, it took two people to carry them. I was in heaven, and that was a migraine-diet cheat day that will live in infamy.) Before this diet, I thought no cheese board was complete without gouda, cheddar, and a stinky blue cheese. It turns out there are a ton of wonderful fresh cheeses. It's all about changing your mindset of how things should be.

CHEESES (PICK 3 OR MORE)

Fresh ricotta

Fresh goat cheese (chèvre)

Fresh, unflavored mozzarella or Oaxaca

Boursin Garlic & Fine Herbs

Cubed deli-style American (Andrew & Everett or Boar's Head)

ACCOMPANIMENTS (PICK 3 OR MORE)

Seeds: sunflower or pepitas (pumpkin seeds)

Pomegranate seeds

Fruits: cherries, grapes, and/or blackberries

Blackberry jam (gelatin- and citrus-free) or honey

Water crackers or migraine-friendly gluten-free crackers (I like Crunchmaster Sea Salt)

GARNISHES (OPTIONAL)

Fresh rosemary, basil, or other herb sprigs, or chopped

Coarse salt and freshly ground black pepper

Select a cheese board or large cutting board. Arrange 3 to 4 cheeses of your choice on the board along with fruit, seeds, and crackers of your choice.

For extra flavor, top the ricotta with pomegranate seeds and spread jam or honey over the goat cheese and top with fresh pepper. Sprinkle mozzarella with coarse salt, fresh basil, and black pepper.

Garnish the platter with fresh herbs and sprinkle the cheese with salt and pepper, if you like.

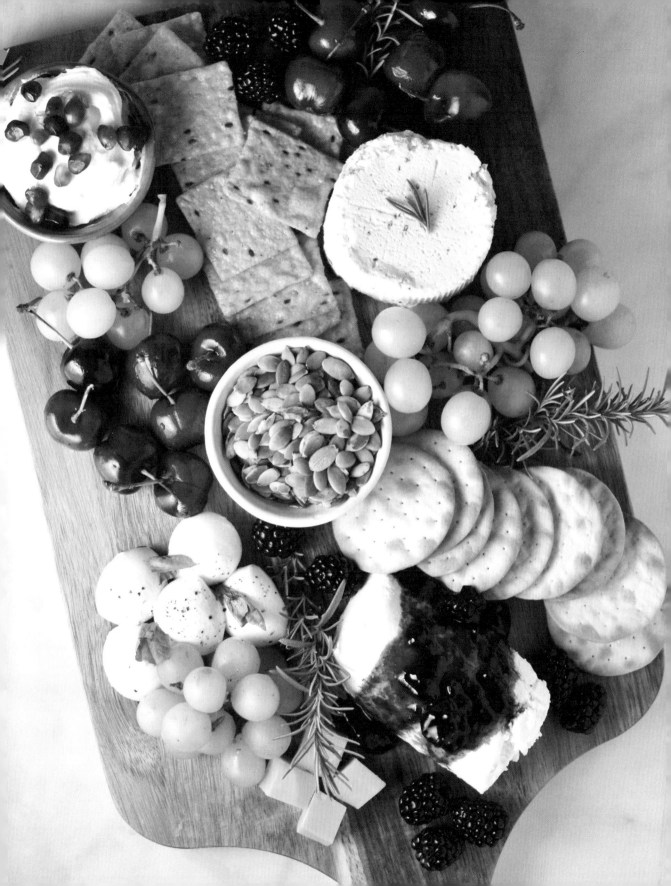

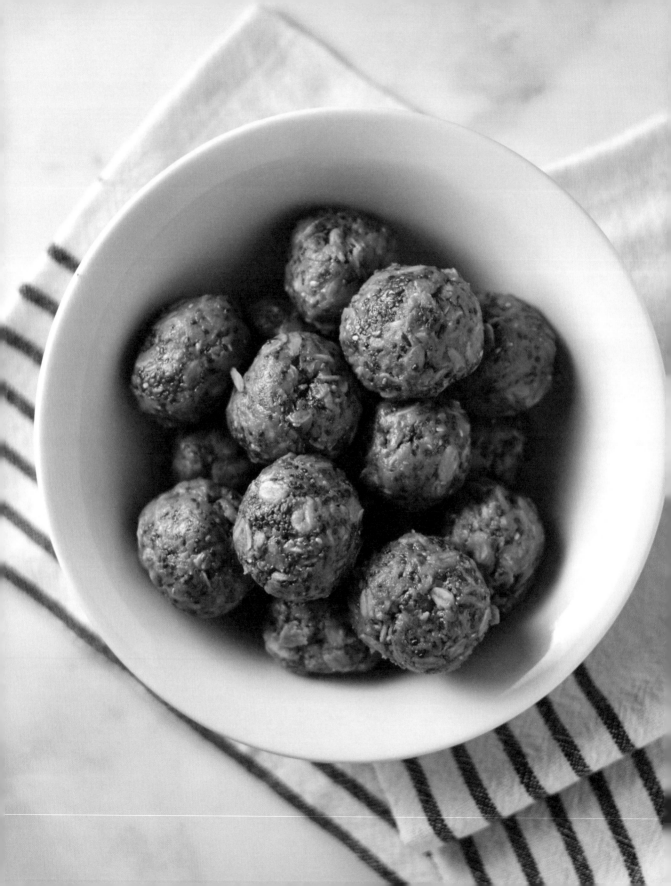

Seed Butter Energy Balls

MAKES 20 BALLS

Great for traveling, perfect for snacks, and packed with protein… what more could you want? These are my go-to snacks for long car trips, plane rides, or even just a quick breakfast on the go. Add a ¼ cup of white chocolate chips for a sweet twist.

1 cup rolled oats (certified gluten-free, if desired), or more if needed

¼ cup flaxseed meal

¼ cup raw pepitas (pumpkin seeds)

1 tablespoon chia seeds

½ cup sunflower seed butter, or more if needed

⅓ cup honey

1 teaspoon vanilla extract

In a medium bowl, combine the oats, flaxseed meal, pepitas, chia seeds, sunflower seed butter, honey, and vanilla. Stir to combine. I then like to use my hands to mush it all together. If the mixture seems too sticky, add more oats. If it seems too dry, add more sunflower seed butter. Cover the mixture and chill for at least 30 minutes.

Form the chilled mixture into 1- to 1½-inch balls and place on a plate. Separate layers with parchment paper. Cover and refrigerate until ready to eat, or put in the freezer for longer storage.

Crispy Taco-Spiced Wings

MAKES 4 TO 6 APPETIZER SERVINGS

I was introduced to this method of cooking wings in baking powder by a food blogger friend and never looked back. Turns out even Serious Eats has a whole article on the chemistry of why this works. Using aluminum-free baking powder (which is important for taste purposes) allows the chicken skin to bubble and also weakens the proteins, so you get a crisp texture without deep-frying. Starting the wings at a low temperature helps the skin to dry out and render the fat. I used my go-to spices for taco night to season these wings and couldn't believe the amount of flavor they had. Dunk them in a little Southwestern Ranch Dressing (page 70) if you really want to go all out. You can also serve these as a main dish for two, accompanied by a big salad like the Maui Kale Salad (page 86) or the Mexican-Style Black Beans (page 187).

---

2 pounds chicken wing segments and/or drumettes

1 tablespoon aluminum-free baking powder

1½ teaspoons kosher salt plus more to taste

Olive oil or olive oil baking spray

½ teaspoon dried oregano

½ teaspoon paprika

½ teaspoon ground cumin

3 cloves garlic, minced

3 tablespoons unsalted butter, melted

Chopped fresh parsley for garnish (optional)

Preheat the oven to 250°F. Spray or rub a wire rack with olive oil and place it over a baking sheet. (You can place aluminum foil on the baking sheet to catch the drippings and make for easy clean-up.)

Thoroughly dry the wings with paper towels and put them in a large bowl. Add the baking powder and salt; toss well. Spread the wings on the rack, making sure they do not touch each other. Bake for 30 minutes.

After 30 minutes, increase the oven heat to 425°F and bake wings until the skin is brown and crispy, flipping halfway through, another 60 minutes.

In a clean large bowl, mix together the oregano, paprika, and cumin. Add the cooked chicken wings, garlic, and melted butter, then toss everything together until evenly coated. Add more salt to taste and serve warm, sprinkled with parsley, if desired.

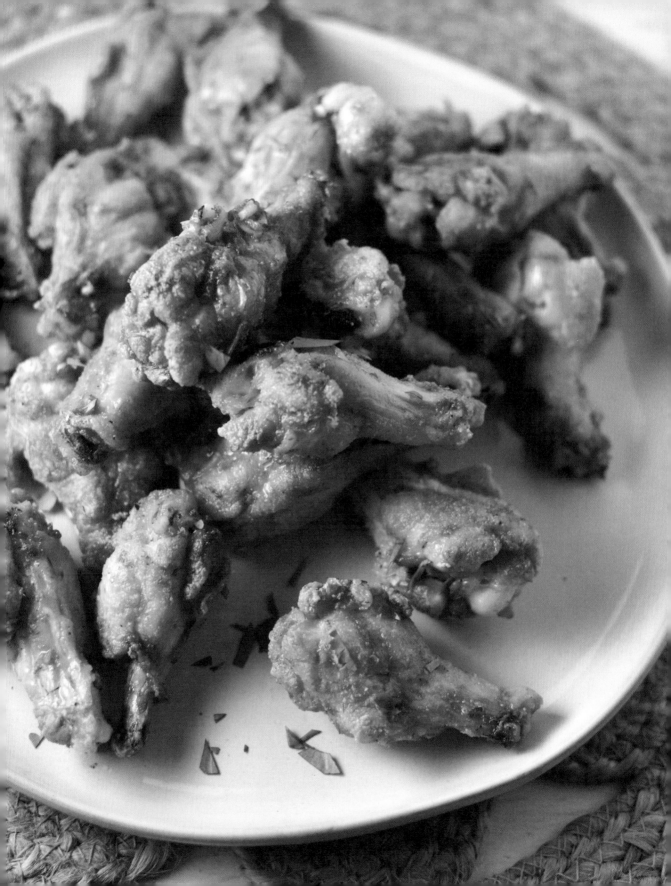

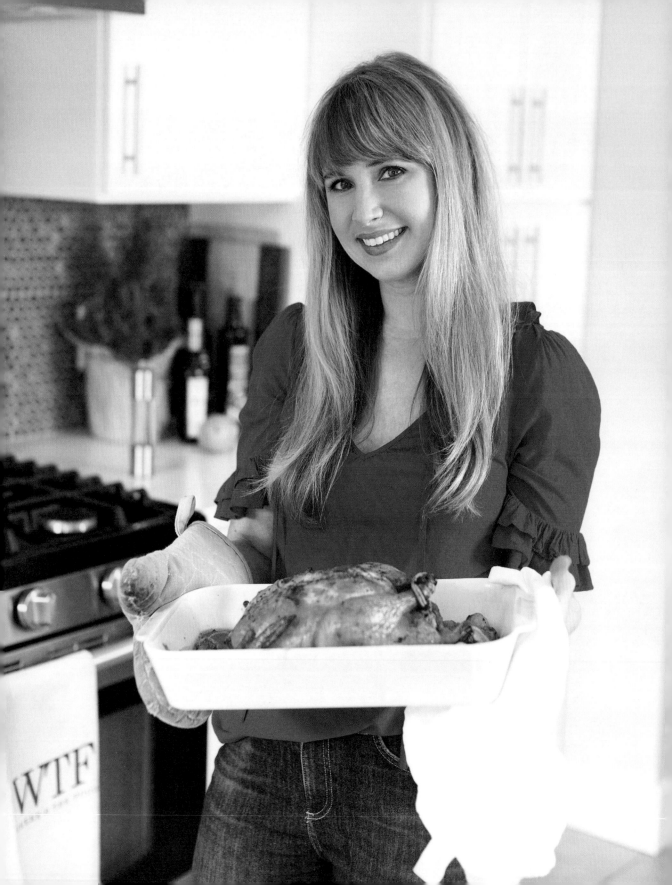

Main Dishes

For this chapter, I wanted to give you main-dish options that will appeal to your entire family. As I said earlier, the more you can get your family on board, the easier it is to follow this diet well. With these comforting recipes, family members won't even notice they're secretly following a migraine-friendly diet! The Salsa Verde Chicken Enchiladas, Mini Barbecue Meatloaves, and Healthy-ish Beef Stroganoff are all healthier versions of meals that I remember enjoying as a kid.

While some of the recipes do require some prep time and a little effort, the Sheet Pan Salmon has two options—one which can be made as a quick meal on a high-pain or discomfort day, and another which can be elevated for a date night at home. The Moroccan Meatballs, Slow Cooker or Instant Pot Pulled Pork, Anyone-Can-Cook Roast Chicken, and Mini Barbecue Meatloaves are simple to prep and freeze to keep on hand when you feel miserable.

Many of the recipes, including the Pumpkin Sage Pasta, Mediterranean-Style Baked Halibut, Roasted Chicken Thighs with Grapes and Brussels Sprouts, Lamb Chops with Cilantro Chimichurri, Seared Sea Scallops with Mango Salsa, and more, can all be made in 30 minutes or less. These dishes are perfect when you're not feeling your best—but also when you are, and you just want to get a quick dinner on the table so that you can go out and have fun.

These recipes are not meant to be intimidating, even though I was very intimidated by my first whole roasted chicken! They're meant to inspire you to realize your full potential as a home cook who also has the added challenge of a migraine disorder. I was at a very low point where cooking seemed too exhausting for me, yet once I forced myself to dive in, I found mindfulness and healing in the process. I even found a little bit of vestibular therapy while looking from one ingredient to the next and carefully moving plates and dishes. But the best thing I discovered was a reconnection to my family that even my migraine disorder couldn't take away. Sitting down and sharing a meal together put the pain further back in my mind, and for that moment it was just us and some really good food. I hope that you will find the same healing through your cooking too.

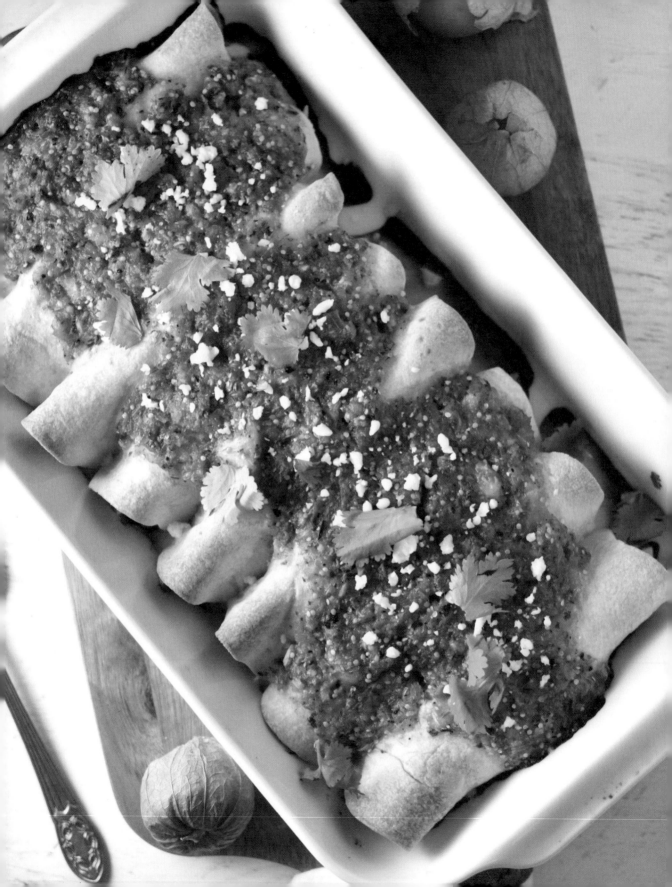

Salsa Verde Chicken Enchiladas

MAKES 4 SERVINGS

The ultimate crowd-pleaser, this recipe is a winner that can be customized in so many ways. To make it vegetarian, substitute zucchini, summer squash, corn, spinach, and/or roasted sweet potatoes for the chicken. Other times it's wonderful with ground beef, using my Enchilada Sauce (page 79) instead of the salsa verde. If you're gluten free, you'll want to use 100 percent corn tortillas (avoid tortillas that use a mix of wheat). If you find that the corn tortillas are breaking while you assemble, wrap them in a damp paper towel and microwave in 30-second increments. Serve these enchiladas with a simple side salad, Mexican-Style Black Beans (page 187), and/or rice.

Olive oil

¾ cup fresh or frozen corn kernels

3 green onions, chopped

1 clove garlic, minced

2 cups chopped cooked chicken ("naked" rotisserie chicken works well here)

1–2 cups chopped kale or spinach

1 teaspoon kosher salt

1 teaspoon ground cumin

½ teaspoon dried oregano

4 ounces cream cheese (carrageenan-free)

8–10 flour or corn tortillas

Charred Salsa Verde (page 83)

Queso fresco and cilantro leaves for garnish (optional)

Preheat the oven to 425°F. Lightly oil an 11-by-17-inch baking dish.

In a large skillet, warm a small amount of olive oil over medium heat. Add the corn, green onions, and garlic; sauté until softened, about 2 minutes. Add the chicken, kale, salt, cumin, and oregano; sauté until the kale wilts down. Remove from heat and mix in the cream cheese until fully incorporated.

Lay the tortillas flat on a work surface. Spoon the filling mixture in a strip down the center of the tortillas, dividing evenly. Roll the tortillas around the filling, placing them seam side down into the prepared baking dish. Pour the Charred Salsa Verde across the middle section of the filled tortillas. I like to leave the ends bare so they get nice and crispy. Bake until bubbling with browned edges, about 20 minutes.

Let the enchiladas cool slightly before serving. If desired, garnish with crumbled queso fresco and cilantro leaves.

> **HEAD-FRIENDLY TORTILLAS** The best place to locate good, migraine-safe tortillas is in the refrigerated section of the grocery store. They typically won't have all the additives that the ones on the shelf will and are more likely to be HYH compliant.

Moroccan Meatballs

MAKES 4 SERVINGS

One of the most popular recipes on my website uses five spices—paprika, cumin, ginger, turmeric, and cinnamon—as a marinade for a simply grilled chicken breast. I wanted to transform it into something that can be more easily frozen and reheated, since many of us don't always know how we will feel when it comes to making dinner. Meatballs are the perfect way to do that. You can use ground chicken, lamb, or beef for this recipe—all with great results. If you use chicken, I find ground chicken thighs are the most flavorful. Gluten-free panko is easy to find. My favorite is Jeff Nathan Creations. Serve this with Pomegranate Couscous (page 179) and an easy, light salad.

---

2 cloves garlic, minced

2 teaspoons paprika

1 teaspoon ground cumin

1 teaspoon kosher salt

¼ teaspoon ground ginger

¼ teaspoon ground turmeric

¼ teaspoon ground cinnamon

3–4 tablespoons olive oil, plus more for cooking, divided

1½ pounds ground chicken, lamb, or beef

¼ cup panko (gluten-free, if desired)

Chopped fresh parsley for garnish (optional)

Preheat the oven to 400°F.

In a large bowl, combine the garlic, paprika, cumin, salt, ginger, turmeric, cinnamon, and 1 tablespoon of the olive oil; stir thoroughly. Add the ground chicken and panko, then mix together with your hands until well combined. Form the mixture into 1½-inch balls. If the mixture isn't sticking together well (this can happen with ground chicken), give it a few minutes in the fridge to firm up.

In a large skillet, warm the remaining 2 to 3 tablespoons olive oil over medium heat. Add the meatballs to the pan, being careful not to overcrowd them. You may need to do this in batches. Cook until the meatballs are browned on each side, about 1 minute per side, then transfer to a baking sheet. Bake until cooked through, about 10 minutes. Serve warm sprinkled with fresh parsley, if desired, or let cool and refrigerate or freeze for later.

To reheat after freezing, preheat the oven to 300°F. Place the meatballs on a baking sheet and cover with foil. Bake for 15 to 18 minutes, until heated through.

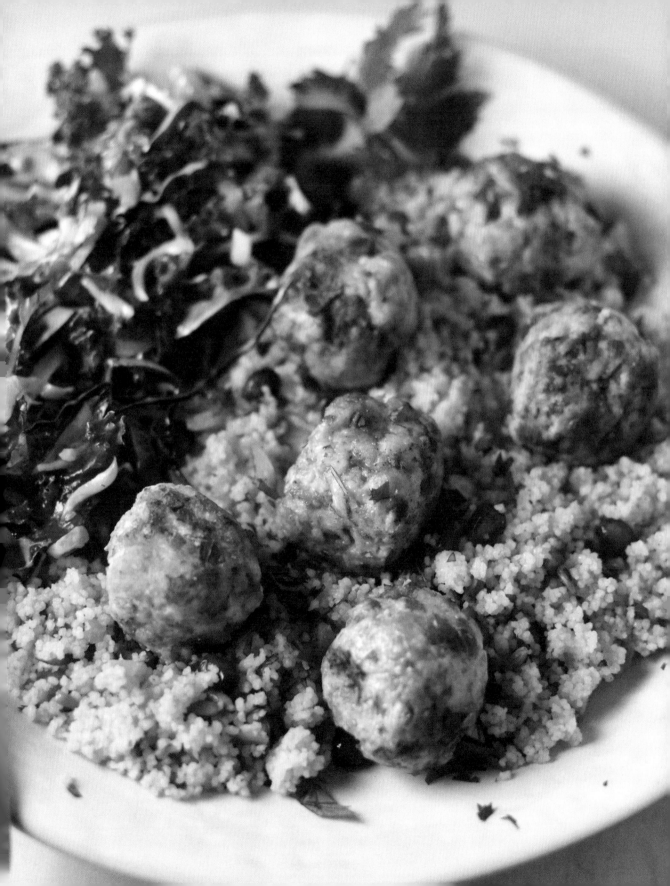

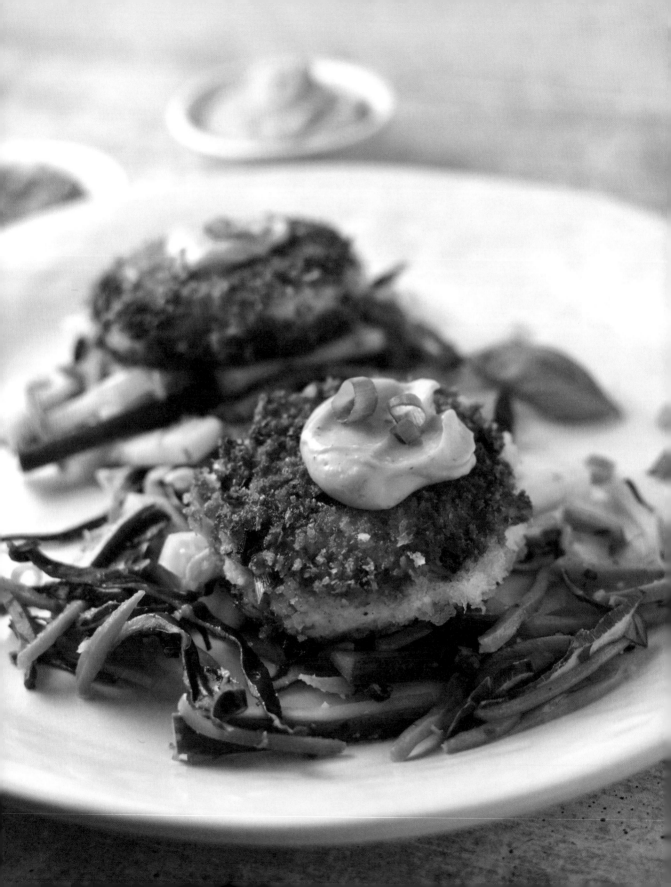

Banh Mi–Inspired Crab Cakes

MAKES 4 SERVINGS

An Asian-flavored meal can be difficult to achieve on a migraine diet, especially without the ability to use fish sauce or soy sauce. Pre-diagnosis, banh mi—Vietnamese-style sandwiches—were one of my favorite items to order at restaurants, so I wanted to get as close as I could to recreating those flavors with head-friendly ingredients. These crab cakes are an easy, full meal with the refreshing cucumber and carrot salad. Don't skip the spicy mayo—it's a must.

16 ounces fresh lump crabmeat

3 tablespoons migraine-friendly mayonnaise

2 tablespoons all-purpose flour (rice flour for gluten-free)

4 green onions, chopped

½ teaspoon kosher salt

1 cup panko breadcrumbs (gluten-free, if desired)

¼ cup neutral cooking oil

HERBED VEGETABLE SALAD

2 tablespoons distilled white vinegar

2 tablespoons chopped fresh basil

2 teaspoons chopped fresh mint

2 teaspoons minced fresh ginger

2 teaspoons toasted sesame oil

2 teaspoons honey

½ teaspoon kosher salt

1 cup shredded cabbage

1 cup *each* matchstick-cut carrots and English cucumber

SPICY MAYO

2 tablespoons migraine-friendly mayonnaise

2 teaspoons Sriracha (sulfite-, citrus-, and MSG-free) or hot sauce

To make the crab cake mixture, pick the crabmeat free of shells. In a large bowl, combine the crabmeat, mayonnaise, flour, green onions (set aside a few pieces for garnish), and salt. Mix with your hands until everything is evenly distributed. Chill for 30 minutes or more, until mixture sticks together well; the colder the mixture is, the better it will hold together. Form the cold mixture into 8 patties, each about 2 to 3 inches in diameter. Place on a plate. Chill until ready to fry.

While the crab cake mixture is chilling, make the salad: In a large bowl, mix together the vinegar, basil, mint, ginger, sesame oil, honey, and salt. Add the cabbage, carrots, and cucumber, and toss well; set aside.

Next, prepare the Spicy Mayo: In a small bowl, mix together mayonnaise and Sriracha. Cover and refrigerate until ready to use.

When you're ready to fry, pour the panko into a large dish. Remove the crab cakes from the refrigerator and coat each patty with panko on both sides, patting gently until it adheres. If you find that they're falling apart, chill the mixture for a little longer.

In a large nonstick skillet, warm the cooking oil over medium heat. Working in batches if necessary, carefully add the panko-coated crab cakes to the pan, which should sizzle when they contact the oil. Cook for 4 minutes on the first side, flip, then another 3 minutes. You want them to be nicely browned on both sides. Drain the crab cakes on a paper towel, then transfer to a 200°F oven to keep warm while you fry the remaining crab cakes.

Divide the salad among 4 plates, then place 2 crab cakes on top of each. Serve with the Spicy Mayo and the reserved green onion pieces.

Sheet Pan Salmon, Kale & Potatoes with Dijon-Dill Sauce

MAKES 4 SERVINGS

Technically, the salmon, kale, and potatoes all cook on one pan (yay, fewer dishes to wash!), but you must use an additional pan for the cream sauce (boo, she tricked us!). If you just don't have the energy to make the sauce, this dinner is healthy and flavorful with simply seasoned salmon. I adored sheet pan meals in my early days of chronic VM—the less I had to deal with, the better. If it's a good day for you and you are feeling up to it, the sauce really elevates the meal and makes it feel decadent. When buying butter and cream, be sure to avoid "natural flavors" and additives like carrageenan.

SALMON, KALE & POTATOES

1½ pounds fingerling potatoes, halved lengthwise

Olive oil

Kosher salt and freshly ground black pepper

1 large bunch lacinato (dinosaur) kale

1½ pounds fresh salmon fillets

DIJON-DILL SAUCE

1 tablespoon unsalted butter

1 very small shallot, minced (about 1½ tablespoons)

¾ cup Vegetable Broth (page 80) or Chicken Stock (page 81)

1½ tablespoons Dijon mustard (wine- and sulfite-free)

¼ cup heavy cream (carrageenan free)

1 tablespoon chopped fresh dill

Preheat the oven to 425°F. Cover a large baking sheet with parchment paper. Put the potatoes on the baking sheet along with 1 tablespoon olive oil, and salt and pepper to taste. Stir to combine, then roast for 15 minutes.

Meanwhile, wash the kale, spin it dry, and remove the coarse stalks by sliding your knife along each side of the rib. Tear the kale leaves into 2- to 3-inch pieces. Pat the salmon dry on both sides.

Remove the potatoes from the oven and toss them around. Reduce the oven heat to 400°F. Nestle the salmon fillets, skin side down, and kale among the potatoes on the baking sheet. Rub a little bit of olive oil on top of the salmon and throughout the kale. Sprinkle everything with a little salt and pepper. Roast until the salmon is almost cooked through and the kale is brown and crispy, another 15 minutes.

To make the Dijon-Dill Sauce, melt the butter in a medium saucepan over medium heat. Add the shallot and sauté for 1 minute. Add the broth or stock, bring to a simmer, and cook until reduced by about half, about 5 minutes. Stir in the mustard and cream, then continue to barely simmer for another 3 minutes. The sauce should be thick enough that when you slide a wooden spoon through it, it leaves a little trail. Sprinkle in the chopped fresh dill.

To serve, divide the salmon, potatoes, and kale among serving plates and top the salmon with the sauce. Serve warm.

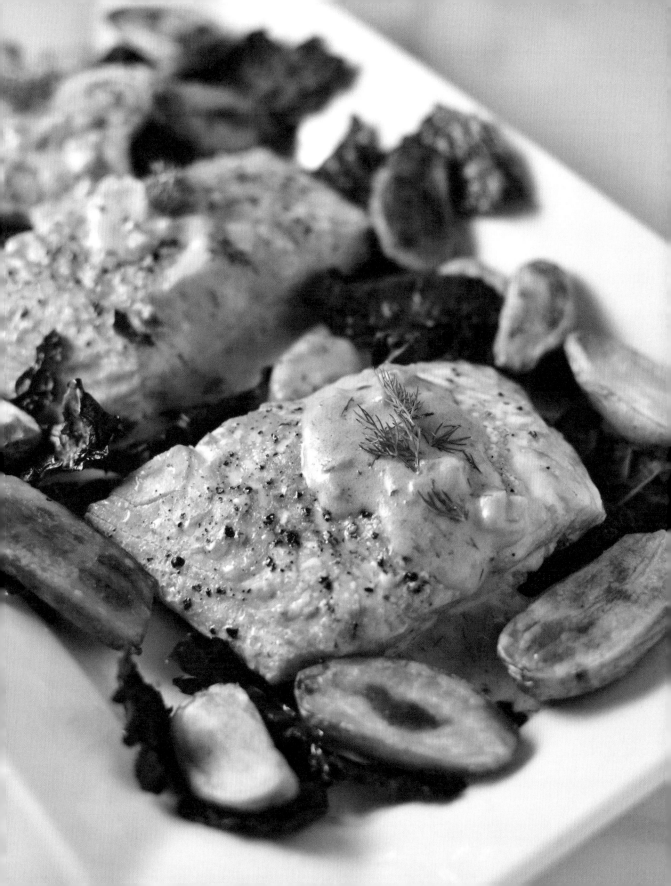

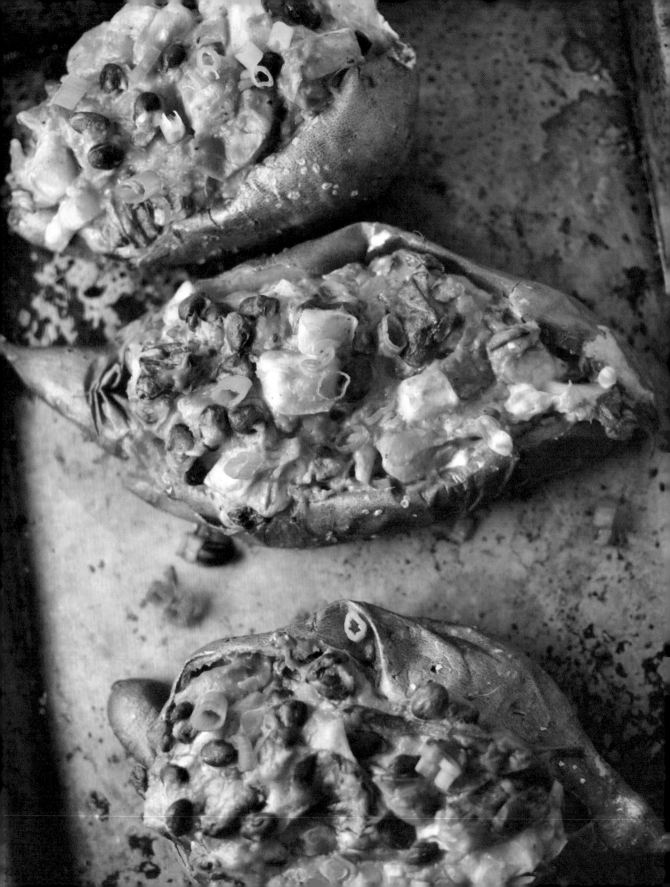

Mexican-Style Stuffed Sweet Potatoes

MAKES 4 SERVINGS

My husband might keel over if I ever decided to go on strictly plant-based diet, but I do like to eat that way at least a couple nights a week. Focusing on vegetables allows you to get a little more creative with meals. These potatoes take time to cook but are well worth it. Coming from someone whose love for cheese knows no bounds, I really don't miss it in this recipe. The sweet potato filling provides creaminess and the spicy sauce packs a ton of flavor.

4 sweet potatoes of a similar size, scrubbed clean and dried

2 tablespoons extra-virgin olive oil, divided

Kosher salt and freshly ground black pepper

1 small summer squash, cut into ½-inch pieces

1 shallot, minced

7–8 ounces canned black beans, drained (about half of a 15-ounce can)

1 cup fresh spinach

Enchilada Sauce (page 79)

2 green onions, chopped

Preheat oven to 400°F.

Take a fork and poke a few holes all over the sweet potatoes. Place them on a baking sheet, drizzle with 1 tablespoon olive oil and some salt, and bake until soft all the way through, 50 to 60 minutes. (If you haven't already, you can make the Enchilada Sauce while the sweet potatoes are cooking.)

Once the sweet potatoes are done, take them out of the oven but keep the oven heated to 400°F. Cut a slit in the top of the sweet potatoes lengthwise and scoop out some of the filling, leaving a place for you to put the filling. Set aside the scooped-out sweet potato.

In a large skillet, warm the remaining 1 tablespoon olive oil over medium heat. Add the squash and shallot; sauté until slightly browned, 2 to 4 minutes. Add the black beans, scooped-out sweet potato, and spinach. Cook until mixture is warmed through and spinach is slightly wilted, another 2 minutes. Stir in ⅓ cup of the Enchilada Sauce.

Scoop the vegetable mixture into each hollowed-out sweet potato, dividing evenly. Place back in the oven until heated through, another 15 minutes. Top each potato with extra sauce (you may not use all of it) and the chopped green onions. Serve immediately.

Mini Barbecue Meatloaves

MAKES 6 MINI MEATLOAVES.

Earlier in the book, I mentioned how my approach to cooking is a little bit different from other migraine diet resources. Elimination diets are hard, and you already feel like you're giving up a lot in other areas of your life just to manage this illness. That's why I believe having comfort food is so important, while still being healthy and eliminating triggers. Just making the switch from pre-packaged barbecue sauce to making your own is a big step in taking control of your health. Here, I use it to coat individual meatloaves for a homestyle meal everyone will love. Pair them with the Whipped Parsnips (page 183) or simple mashed potatoes for a complete meal, or with a tossed green salad for something lighter.

---

1 pound ground beef

⅓ cup rolled oats (certified gluten-free, if desired)

1 large egg, lightly beaten

1 shallot, chopped

1 clove garlic, minced

1 teaspoon minced fresh parsley, plus more for garnish (optional)

½ teaspoon dried oregano

½ teaspoon kosher salt

Barbecue Sauce (page 75)

Preheat the oven to 400°F. Line a baking sheet with parchment paper.

In a large bowl, combine the ground beef, oats, egg, shallot, garlic, parsley, oregano, and salt. Mix with your hands until just combined.

Divide the meat into 6 portions. Gently form each portion into a loaf shape, place on the prepared baking sheet, and flatten slightly, separating the loaves from each other on the pan. Using a spoon, top each loaf with a dollop of Barbecue Sauce and spread it to the edges. Bake the loaves until the sauce has set on top and the meatloaves are just cooked through, about 20 minutes. Serve warm garnished with minced parsley, if desired, with extra sauce on the side.

> **TOMATO TROUBLE** If you cannot tolerate the tomatoes in the Barbecue Sauce, you can make these meatloaves into meatballs instead. Serve them with pasta or on top of a salad. Or, try using a "nomato" sauce, which is typically made from beets and carrots.

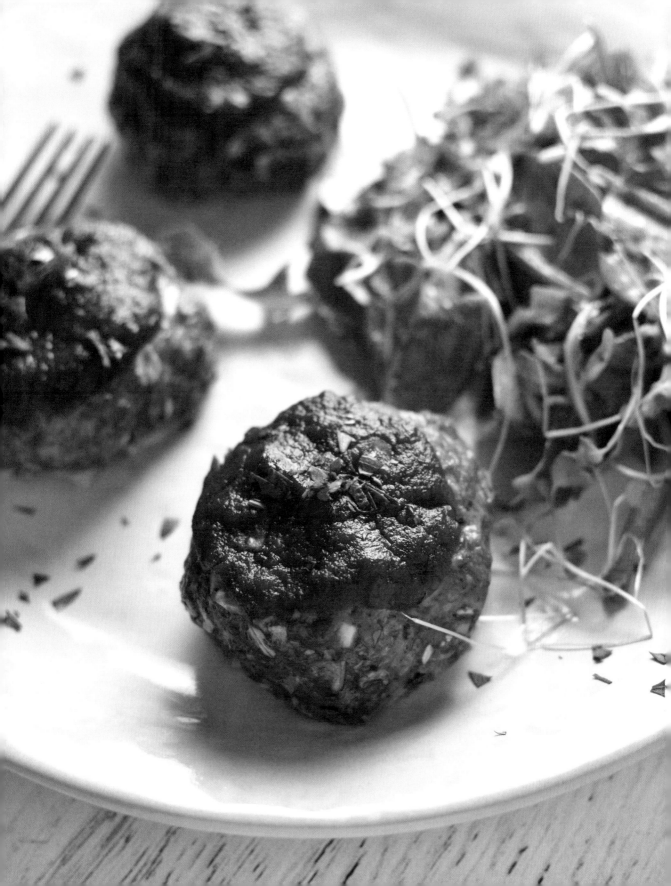

Anyone-Can-Cook Roast Chicken with Rosemary Gravy

MAKES 4 SERVINGS

Believe it or not, a roasted chicken is one of the easiest things you can make. I used to be one of those people who thought it would be a huge hassle, until I tried it! You may recognize the name from one of my favorite movies, *Ratatouille*. The overall theme is that an excellent cook can come from the most unlikely places… perhaps someone with chronic migraine? My first time testing this recipe I was in the middle of an attack. Powering through, I stuffed my chicken with aromatics and carefully placed it into the roasting pan. It came out gorgeous and lightly brown in all the right places. I was so proud of myself, I took the pictures to share my accomplishment with everyone. Then my husband walked over and asked why it was upside down. It wasn't perfect, but it was delicious! The lemongrass stalks add a nice scent of lemon without the citrus. I like to serve this with Mac & Fresh Cheese (page 175) and Asparagus with Fresh Dill Vinaigrette (page 176). Adding assorted root vegetables like carrots, radishes, or turnips to the roasting pan can provide a quick and easy side dish as well.

ROAST CHICKEN

1 whole chicken, about 4 pounds

2 lemongrass stalks

1 bunch fresh thyme or lemon thyme (if you can find it) sprigs

4 cloves garlic (2 whole and 2 sliced), divided

2 tablespoons unsalted butter, at room temperature

1 tablespoon olive oil

4 large shallots, quartered

¾ pound assorted small root vegetables, cut into chunks (optional)

Kosher salt and freshly ground black pepper

Preheat oven to 425°F. Find a roasting pan that's large enough for the chicken, but not too large that the shallots and vegetables will burn. You want to have just a little bit of space directly around the chicken.

Pat the chicken dry with paper towels; reach up into the cavity and pull out any bags of giblets that you sometimes find there.

Remove the woody ends from the lemongrass by cutting right where the white turns more green. Throw away the ends and cut the stalk into 3-inch pieces, then halve each piece lengthwise. Smash each stalk once or twice with the wide section of your knife to release some of the lemon scent. Stuff it in the chicken cavity along with a small handful of the fresh thyme sprigs and the 2 whole garlic cloves.

Starting at the leg cavity, carefully slide your fingers just under the chicken skin, loosening it from the flesh over the breasts and the legs. Rub the softened butter under the chicken skin and place the sliced garlic under the skin. Finally, rub 1 tablespoon olive oil all over the outside of the skin.

ROSEMARY GRAVY

Pan drippings from roasting
the chicken

1 tablespoon unsalted butter,
ghee, or olive oil

1 tablespoon all-purpose flour,
sweet rice flour, or white rice
flour

1 cup Chicken Stock (page 81)
or Vegetable Broth
(page 80)

1 teaspoon chopped fresh
rosemary

1 teaspoon chopped fresh
thyme

Place the chicken in the roasting pan, breast side up, and tie the legs together with kitchen twine. Arrange the shallots and root vegetables (if using) around the chicken. Sprinkle everything with kosher salt and pepper. Roast until the chicken's internal temperature reaches 165°F when an instant-read thermometer is inserted into the largest part of the thigh, away from the bone, about 1 hour and 5 minutes.

Transfer the chicken and shallots to a cutting board, then cover with foil to keep warm.

To make the Rosemary Gravy, scrape the drippings from the roasting pan into a medium skillet and add the butter. Over medium heat, whisk in the flour until it turns a nice caramel brown color. Add in the stock a little bit at a time, whisking after each addition until smooth. Simmer for about 5 minutes until it becomes a thicker gravy-like consistency. Whisk in the rosemary and thyme.

To serve, parade that beautiful bird around in front of your family like the expert cook you are, then carve the meat on a cutting board (it helps to have one with slats around the edges to catch the juices). It's best to start by removing the legs first, then make a long cut down the base of the chicken to begin to remove the breasts. Hold your chicken near the breastbone (a large fork can help), then slide your knife down each side to remove the breasts. Serve the meat warm with a side of the gravy, or just pour the gravy on top.

A MIGRAINE KITCHEN WORKHORSE Additive-free cooked chicken is hard to find, but you can easily make your own for countless recipes using this recipe as your base. Omit the shallots, root vegetables, and gravy, and this makes a great staple recipe to use in lunches or for the White Bean Chicken Chili (page 105), Farro & Lemongrass Chicken Soup (page 109), or Salsa Verde Chicken Enchiladas (page 137). Pick the meat from the carcass and freeze what you don't think you'll eat right away. Use the carcass to make Chicken Stock (page 81).

Pumpkin Sage Pasta

MAKES 2 SERVINGS

Like a healthy mac & cheese but with an autumnal spin to it, this dish is a quick meal that you can make with mostly pantry staples. One of my favorite parts is the texture that comes from the crunchy toasted pepitas on top. With the sage mixed in, it's such a cozy flavor profile that feels more decadent than it is. (Use 1 teaspoon of dried sage leaves if you forget to buy fresh.) We eat this pasta almost weekly in the fall and winter. A nice substitute for pumpkin would be butternut squash or even mashed sweet potato. My favorite type of pasta to use is zucchette, if you can find it. They look like little pumpkins! Orecchiette is another great alternative—little bowls that scoop up the delicious sauce. A tossed green salad with 1-2-3 Dressing (page 71) would round out the meal simply.

½ pound pasta of choice
(I used trottole here)

2 tablespoons unsalted butter

1 medium shallot, minced

1 clove garlic, minced

½ (15-ounce) can unflavored
pumpkin puree

1 ounce unflavored cream
cheese (carrageenan-free)
or fresh goat cheese (chèvre)

1 tablespoon chopped fresh
sage, plus leaves for garnish
(if desired)

Kosher salt and freshly ground
black pepper

¼ cup pepitas (pumpkin seeds),
toasted

2 tablespoons chopped fresh
chives

Bring a large pot of salted water to a boil and cook the pasta according to its package directions. Reserve 1 cup of the cooking water, then drain the pasta. Do not rinse.

Meanwhile, in a large skillet, melt the butter over medium heat. Add the shallot and garlic and sauté until fragrant, about 2 minutes. Then add the pumpkin puree and stir to combine. Add ¼ cup of the reserved pasta water at a time until desired consistency is reached. Whisk in the cream cheese and sage until creamy and thick. Add the hot pasta and toss to coat well. Season with salt and pepper to taste.

Divide the pasta among serving dishes and top with the toasted pepitas, chives, and sage leaves (if using). Serve immediately.

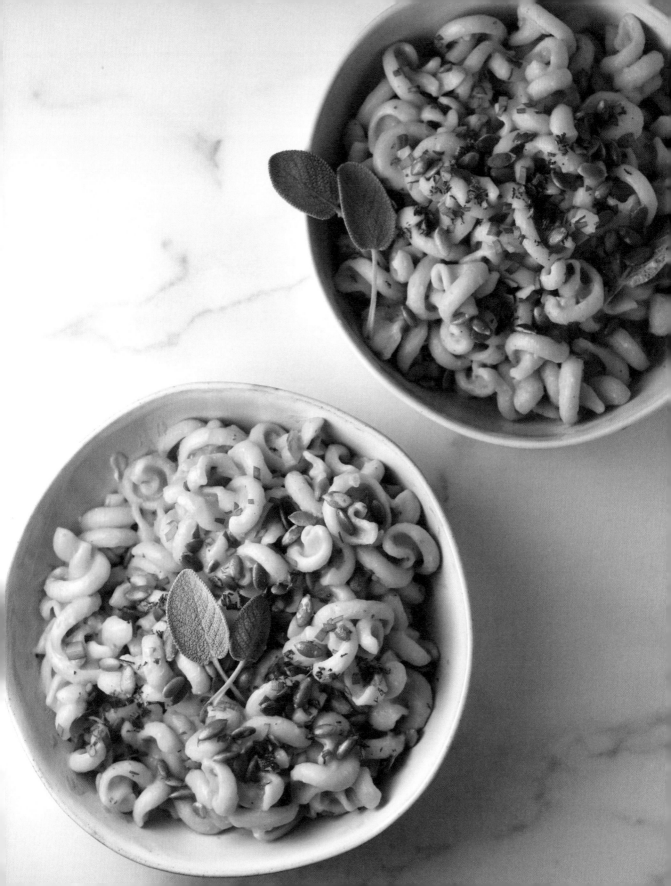

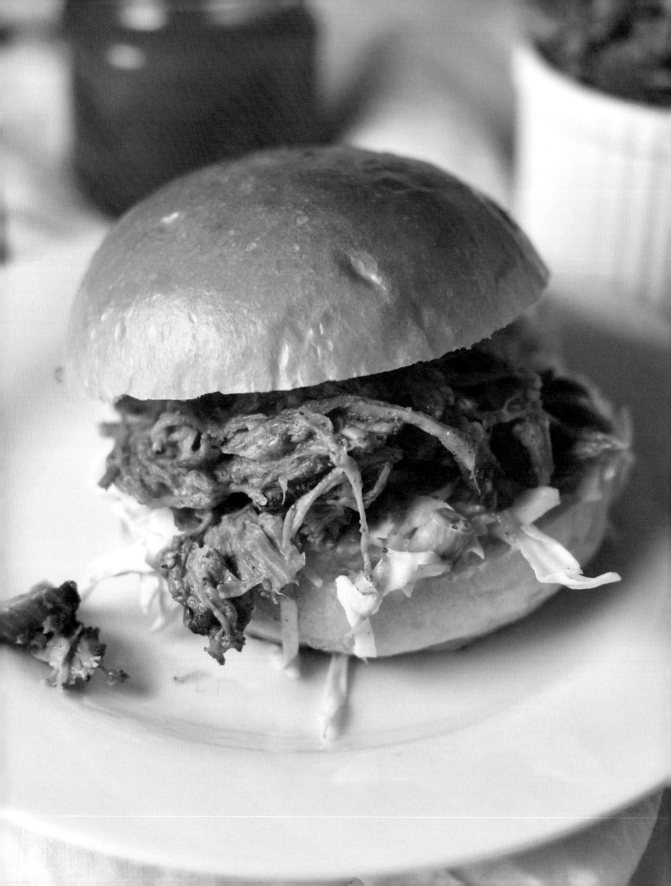

Slow Cooker or Instant Pot Pulled Pork

MAKES 6 TO 8 SERVINGS

This is another great recipe for those days where minimal effort is desired. Dump everything into the slow cooker, wait a few hours, and it comes out flavorful and delicious. Pulled pork is incredibly versatile. Fry it up with some eggs for breakfast; tuck it into enchiladas or sandwiches for lunch or dinner; put it on top of a salad or baked potato, or inside a tortilla with some American or Oaxacan cheese for a quesadilla. Pulled pork freezes beautifully, so if you want to make a big batch on Sunday, you can have it ready to go for the rest of the week or be prepared for if/when a migraine attack strikes. For barbecue pork sandwiches, serve this on burger buns with the Barbecue Sauce on page 75. You can use bone-in pork shoulder; it will just take a little bit longer to cook.

---

3 shallots, sliced

4 cloves garlic, sliced

1–2 cups Chicken Stock (page 81) or Vegetable Broth (page 80)

1 tablespoon brown sugar or maple syrup

1 tablespoon chili powder

1 teaspoon ground cumin

½ teaspoon ground cinnamon

3½–4 pounds boneless pork shoulder, netting removed

Kosher salt

To cook with a slow cooker: Place the shallots and garlic in the slow cooker, then add 1 cup stock. In a bowl, combine the brown sugar or maple syrup, chili powder, cumin, and cinnamon, then pat on all sides of the pork. Place it on top of the shallots and garlic. Cover the slow cooker and cook the pork on high for 6 to 8 hours, or on low for 8 to 10 hours. The meat should shred easily with a fork when done. Remove the meat from the liquid and use a fat skimmer or separator to remove the fat from the sauce. You can return the shredded meat and de-fatted sauce to the slow cooker and keep on warm. Season with salt.

To cook with an Instant Pot: Cut the pork shoulder into 4 large chunks. In a bowl, combine the brown sugar or maple syrup, chili powder, cumin, and cinnamon, then pat on all sides of the pork. Add the pork to the Instant Pot and add 2 cups of stock. Following the manufacturer's instructions, lock the lid and set to pressure cook for 50 minutes. Once time is up, allow the pot to release naturally by not touching it for another 15 minutes. Release the valve to allow any excess steam to escape and open the lid. You can turn on the sauté option to reduce some of the liquid. Season with salt.

> SMART TOOL The Instant Pot is a great tool to have on hand for migraine sufferers because the quick-cooking method helps avoid tyramine buildup in meats, but I think you lose a lot of flavor that you get from cooking longer in a slow cooker. Still, it's always nice to have a backup plan if you forget to start a long-cooking braise ahead of time.

Mediterranean-Style Baked Halibut

MAKES 2 TO 3 SERVINGS

An under-20-minute meal that's healthy and has minimal ingredients? Sign me up! This one was inspired by the Mediterranean-style fish sandwiches I used to make during the summer. I would combine sun-dried tomatoes with capers, parsley, mayonnaise, and fresh halibut. Some of my best ideas come from when I feel too exhausted to cook. One day, during an attack, instead of mixing the ingredients together in a bowl (except for capers, which are off limits) and waiting for the topping to chill, I just threw everything on top of the fish, baked it in the oven, and hoped for the best. It turned out wonderfully! If you can, find fresh sun-dried tomatoes that don't contain sulfites. I believe those taste better, but the ones packed in oil are fine too. Just make sure to drain them thoroughly and pat them dry. If tomatoes are not well tolerated, omit them from this recipe. Well-paired side dishes include Boursin Scalloped Potatoes (page 188) or roasted potatoes, and Basil Green Bean Salad (page 191).

2–3 tablespoons migraine-friendly mayonnaise

2–3 tablespoons chopped sun-dried tomatoes (sulfite-free)

2 small cloves garlic, minced

1 tablespoon chopped fresh basil

¼ teaspoon dried oregano

Pinch of crushed red pepper flakes

1 pound fresh halibut fillets

Kosher salt and freshly ground black pepper

Chopped fresh parsley for garnish (optional)

Preheat the oven to 425°F. Line a baking sheet with parchment paper.

In a small bowl, mix together the mayonnaise, sun-dried tomatoes, garlic, basil, oregano, and red pepper flakes. Place the fish, skin side down, on the prepared sheet and season lightly with salt and pepper. Spread the garlic-mayo mixture on top of each fillet and bake until just cooked through, 15 to 17 minutes.

Divide the fillets among serving plates. Garnish with parsley, if desired, and serve immediately.

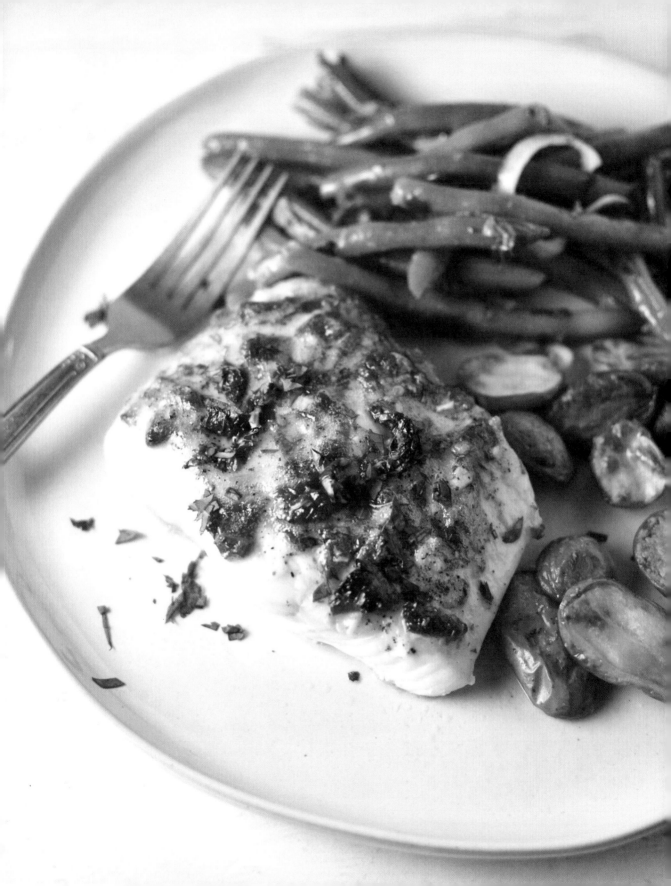

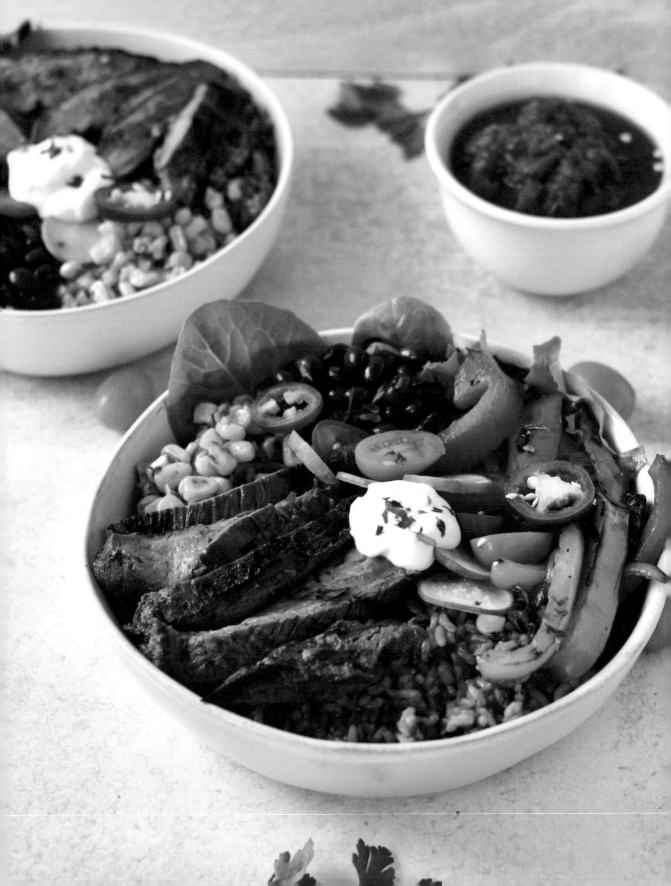

Grilled Chipotle Steak Fajita Bowls

MAKES 4 SERVINGS

I guess now is a bad time to let you know that Chipotle is one of the most migraine-safe fast food chains out there. Hopefully you haven't thrown this book down on the floor as you make a beeline for the door. But if you're looking to make your own chipotle-spiced burrito bowl at home, this is the recipe for you! My secret for the best marinated flank steak is to use tart cherry juice in the marinade. It's a nice substitute for the citrus juices you see in most other recipes, and in my opinion, it tastes even better. You could easily use this meat for tacos if you're not in a bowl mood.

CHIPOTLE STEAK

¼ cup tart cherry juice

2 tablespoons olive oil

1 tablespoon distilled white vinegar

2 cloves garlic, minced

1 teaspoon ground cumin

1 teaspoon chipotle chile powder

1 teaspoon kosher salt

¾ teaspoon dried oregano

1½ pounds flank steak

BOWL COMPONENTS

Shredded or leaf lettuce

Hot cooked cauliflower rice or brown rice

Sautéed bell peppers and shallots

Mexican-Style Black Beans (page 187)

Cooked corn kernels

Crumbled queso fresco

Quick Tomato Salsa or Charred Salsa Verde (page 83)

Chopped fresh cilantro

Sliced jalapeños

To make the Chipotle Steak, in a large locking plastic bag, combine the cherry juice, olive oil, vinegar, garlic, cumin, chipotle powder, salt, and oregano. Score the steak by making very shallow cuts into the meat in a cross-hatch pattern. Place the flank steak inside the bag, moving it around so it's fully coated, and seal the bag. Let the steak marinate for at least 30 minutes or up to 24 hours. (If you're only marinating for 30 minutes, leave it out at room temperature, but if you're marinating for longer, place it in the fridge. The steak should be left out at room temperature for 30 minutes before grilling.)

Preheat the grill to 425–450°F or a grill pan medium-high heat. Remove the steak from the marinade and place it on the grill directly over the heat until well marked with grill marks, about 5 minutes on the first side, then flip and grill for about 5 minutes on the other side for medium-rare. Adjust the cooking time to your liking. Remove the steak from the grill, cover with foil, and allow to rest for about 10 minutes before slicing.

When you're ready to serve, thinly slice the flank steak across the grain. Across the grain is important because it shortens the meat fibers and makes a tougher cut of meat more tender to chew. Build the bowls to your liking, layering your ingredients of choice in the bowls and topping with sliced flank steak.

> **FAUX SOUR CREAM** For a head-friendly creamy element, blend ½ cup cottage cheese (without live cultures) and 1 to 2 teaspoons of distilled white vinegar in a food processor until smooth.

Hearty Wine-Free Short Ribs

MAKES 4 SERVINGS

Finding recipes that don't include red wine (or beer) for braising short ribs is nearly impossible—trust me, I've searched far and wide! One night I decided to try pear juice, fearful the dish might turn out too sweet. But the result was delicious, with only a tiny hint of sweetness. It's amazing how this diet can force us to get creative. Now I prefer this method to the traditional versions with alcohol. I love to serve this on top of Whipped Parsnips (page 183) or mashed potatoes. You can find pear juice at most grocery stores; just make sure it has no added sugar and is not mixed with another type of juice. If you absolutely cannot find a decent pear juice, apple juice is an acceptable substitute.

2 tablespoons olive oil

3–4 pounds bone-in beef short ribs

Kosher salt and freshly ground black pepper

2 celery stalks, chopped

2 large shallots, chopped

2 carrots, chopped

4 cloves garlic, sliced

2 teaspoons dried thyme

1 cup unsweetened pear juice

2 cups Chicken Stock (page 81) or Vegetable Broth (page 80)

Fresh parsley leaves for garnish (optional)

Bring the meat to room temperature 30 minutes before cooking. Preheat the oven to 350°F.

Heat oil in a large Dutch oven over medium-high heat. Season the short ribs with salt and pepper on all sides. When the oil is shimmering but not smoking, add the short ribs and sear until deeply browned, about 2 minutes on the large sides and 1 minute on the small sides. It helps to leave them untouched. You may need to cook them in batches. Set the browned ribs aside on a plate.

Once the ribs are all seared, add the celery, shallots, and carrots to the Dutch oven and sauté until softened, 2 to 3 minutes. Add the garlic and cook another 2 minutes. Finally, add the thyme, juice, and stock or broth.

Bring the mixture to a boil and place the meat back in the pot, trying to get it in a single layer as best as you can. Cover the pot and place in the oven until the meat is very tender and falling off the bone, about 2 hours and 15 minutes.

Transfer the short ribs to a large serving platter. You might need to skim some of the fat off the top of the sauce left in the pot. If desired, simmer the sauce on the stovetop to thicken. Season sauce with salt and pepper to taste, then pour on top of the short ribs. Garnish with parsley leaves, if desired, and serve.

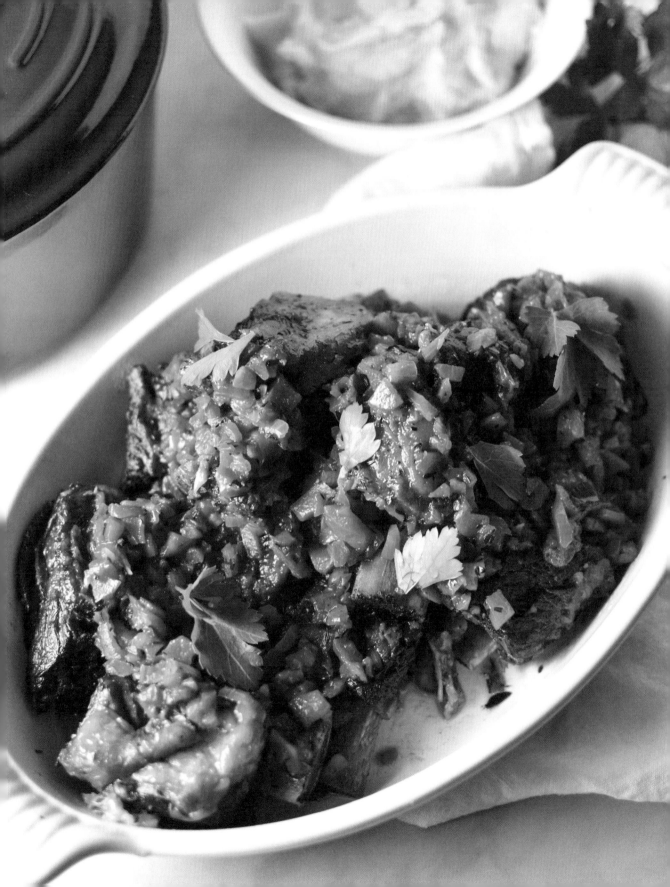

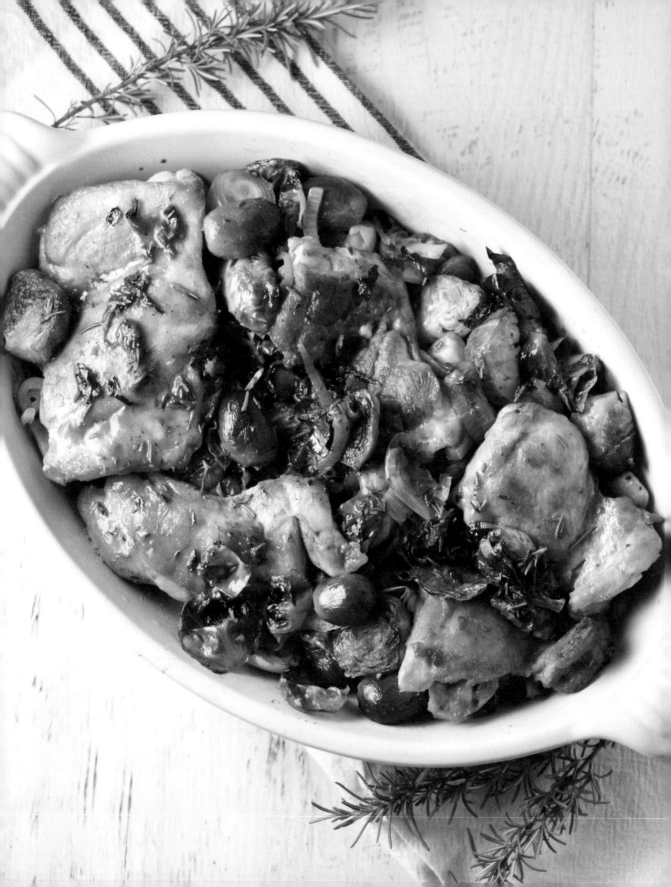

Roasted Chicken Thighs
with Grapes and Brussels Sprouts

MAKES 2 TO 4 SERVINGS

To me there's nothing better than a one-pan meal. You already know I love roasted grapes, based on my Bruschetta Board (page 120), and here they pair well with savory Brussels sprouts for a fresh new twist on chicken dinner.

---

2 tablespoons olive oil

1 pound boneless, skinless chicken thighs

Kosher salt and freshly ground black pepper

1 pound Brussels sprouts, ends trimmed, halved

1 cup seedless red grapes

2 large shallots, thinly sliced

2 tablespoons unsalted butter

1 teaspoon minced fresh rosemary

½ teaspoon dried thyme

½ cup Vegetable Broth (page 80) or Chicken Stock (page 81)

Preheat the oven to 425°F. In a large ovenproof skillet or cast-iron pan, heat the olive oil over medium-high heat. Season the chicken thighs with a little salt and pepper on both sides. When the oil is shimmering, add the chicken thighs and sear until nicely browned on the first side, about 3 minutes, then flip and sear to brown the other side, another 2 to 3 minutes. You may need to do this in batches, so you don't overcrowd the pan, otherwise the chicken will not brown. Transfer the chicken to a plate and set aside.

To the same pan, add the Brussels sprouts. Sauté until lightly browned, about 2 minutes. Add the grapes and browned chicken thighs with any juices from the plate, along with the shallots. Put the pan in the oven and roast until everything is nicely browned and cooked through, about 15 minutes. Remove the pan from the oven.

Transfer the chicken, Brussels sprouts, grapes, and shallots to a deep serving dish (something that can hold a little sauce), leaving behind any pan juices. Protect your hand with an oven mitt while handling the pan (remember, it's hot!). In the same pan you just used for roasting, melt the butter over medium heat. Add the rosemary, thyme, and broth, then turn up the heat to medium-high. Boil until the liquid is reduced by about half. Pour the sauce over the chicken, Brussels sprouts, grapes, and shallots and serve immediately.

Healthy-ish Beef Stroganoff

MAKES 4 SERVINGS

Stroganoff became popular in the US between the '50s and '60s, and many of us are familiar with using the classic cans of cream of mushroom soup that our moms used to make it with. Unfortunately, for someone with migraine, canned soups typically contain MSG and additives, which can be potent triggers and are extremely high in sodium. Sour cream is another potential trigger that's often used in the traditional recipe. My version has a similar creamy texture but without the junk and sodium. I found that goat cheese provides some tanginess that you would miss without the sour cream. Its consistency also holds up better under higher heat than a substitute like cottage cheese. Ground beef just felt easier to me than using steak—one less item to chop. A simple side salad with one of the dressings from pages 68 to 73 is all you need to round out the meal.

---

8 ounces egg noodles (gluten-free, if desired)

2 tablespoons olive oil, divided

1 pound ground beef

2 shallots, chopped

2 cloves garlic, minced

8 ounces cremini mushrooms, sliced

1 tablespoon all-purpose flour (use 2 teaspoons arrowroot powder or cornstarch for gluten-free)

2 cups Vegetable Broth (page 80) or Chicken Stock (page 81)

¾ cup whole milk

3 ounces fresh goat cheese (chèvre)

1 teaspoon kosher salt

¼ teaspoon dried thyme

Freshly ground black pepper

⅓ cup chopped fresh parsley

Bring a large pot of salted water to a boil. Add the egg noodles and cook according to the package directions. Drain and set aside.

Meanwhile, warm 1 tablespoon of olive oil in a large skillet over medium heat. Add the ground beef. Sauté the meat until browned and no pink remains, about 7 minutes, and then drain away any excess fat. Transfer the meat to a plate and set aside.

In the same skillet, warm the remaining 1 tablespoon olive oil over medium heat. Add the shallots and garlic; sauté for 1 minute. Add the mushrooms and sauté until browned, another 3 minutes. Sprinkle in the flour and stir until it coats the mushrooms and shallots. Add the broth and bring to a simmer, stirring everything together until smooth. Simmer until thickened, about 8 minutes. Add the cooked beef, milk, goat cheese, salt, dried thyme, and black pepper to taste. Serve over the warm egg noodles and top with chopped parsley.

> **TAKE CARE WITH MUSHROOMS** All types of wild and cultivated mushrooms are high in natural glutamate, so some people who are extremely sensitive to glutamate cannot tolerate them. There's no need to eliminate them initially, but you may want to be aware of how you feel after eating them. Button mushrooms appear to be the most well tolerated.

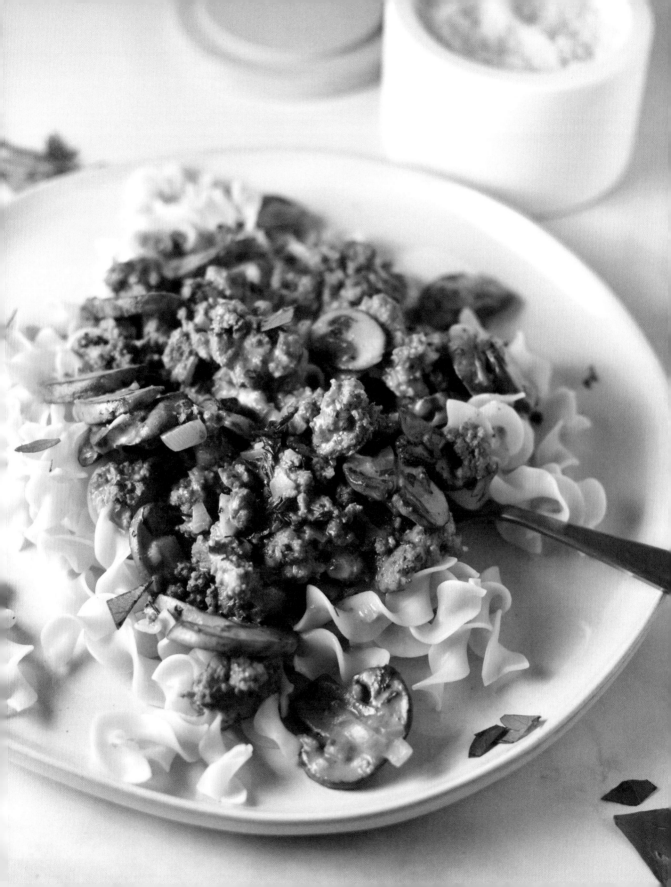

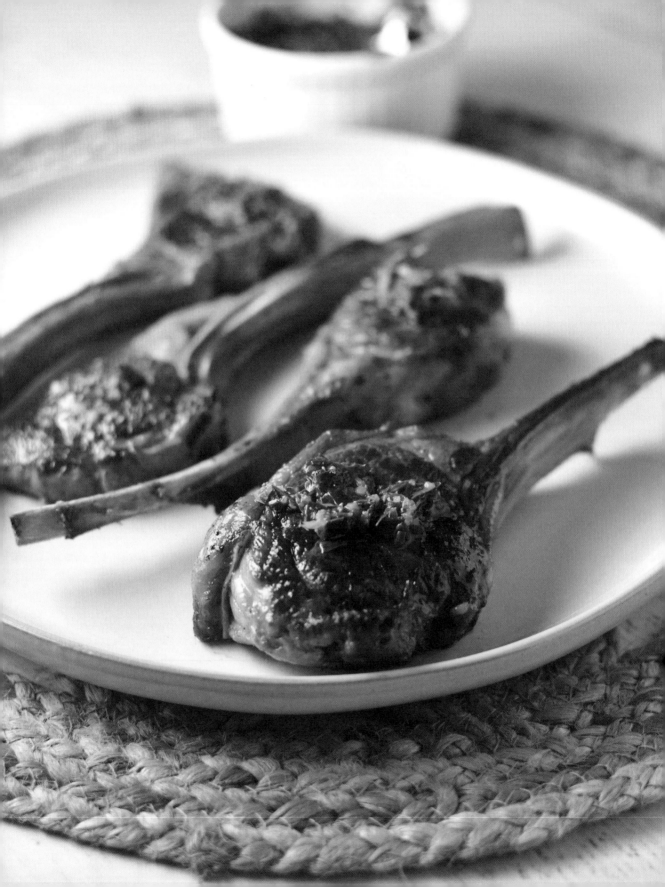

Lamb Chops with Cilantro Chimichurri

MAKES 2 GENEROUS SERVINGS

Craving a date night but don't want to deal with the noise and flickering candles? This is the recipe for you. Sometimes people are intimidated by lamb chops, but in my opinion they're much easier to cook than steak. Seared for just a few minutes on each side, they quickly lead to a gorgeous meal on the table. The chimichurri sauce also works well on seafood, chicken, or steak. This is wonderful with simple roasted potatoes and Garlic Spinach & Tomatoes (page 180).

LAMB CHOPS

1 rack of lamb or about
   2–3 lamb chops per person,
   depending on size, cut into
   individual chops

Kosher salt and freshly ground
   black pepper

2–3 tablespoons olive oil

CILANTRO CHIMICHURRI

1 cup fresh Italian parsley leaves

½ cup fresh cilantro leaves

1 very small shallot

½ clove garlic (add more if you
   want garlic breath for days)

1 teaspoon dried oregano

1 teaspoon crushed red pepper
   flakes

½ teaspoon kosher salt

⅓ cup extra-virgin olive oil

1½ tablespoons distilled white
   vinegar

Pull the lamb chops out of the fridge about 30 minutes before you start cooking.

Meanwhile, make the Cilantro Chimichurri. In a food processor, place the parsley, cilantro, shallot, garlic, oregano, red pepper flakes, salt, ⅓ cup olive oil, and vinegar. Pulse until fully combined, scraping down the sides as needed. Set aside to let the flavors meld.

Sprinkle the lamb chops with salt and black pepper. Heat 2 to 3 tablespoons of olive oil in a large skillet over medium-high heat until shimmering but not smoking. Add the individual lamb chops and sear for 2 to 3 minutes on the first side, until nicely browned. This works best if you just leave it and don't check it until the time is up. Then flip and sear another 2 minutes on the next side for medium-rare. Remove the chops from the pan and cover them with foil. Allow to rest for 10 minutes.

Serve warm with Cilantro Chimichurri on top or on the side.

Seared Sea Scallops with Mango Salsa

MAKES 2 TO 3 SERVINGS

Don't be afraid of scallops—they cook up in less than 5 minutes and are super simple to make if done right. In fact, the most difficult part is purchasing them. Natural scallops are not grey and translucent, they're a milky-white color. You can ask your fishmonger if they've been injected with any solutions. A simple mango salsa makes this a lovely dinner on a warm summer night. You can also use the salsa on chicken or fish tacos. Serve this dish with Charred Corn & Farro Summer Salad (page 89) or a simple side salad with the 1-2-3 Dressing (page 71) for a complete meal.

MANGO SALSA

1 ripe mango, peeled
   and diced

¼ cup fresh cilantro

1 watermelon radish, diced

½ jalapeño chile, seeded
   and minced

1 tablespoon minced shallot

1 teaspoon distilled white
   vinegar

¼ teaspoon sumac

Kosher salt to taste

SEARED SEA SCALLOPS

1 pound large, fresh sea scallops

½ teaspoon curry powder

1 tablespoon unsalted butter

1 tablespoon olive oil

Mixed greens and/or
   microgreens for serving

To make the Mango Salsa, in a small bowl, stir together the mango, cilantro, radish, jalapeño, shallot, vinegar, and sumac. Season to taste with salt. Cover and refrigerate until you're ready to start the scallops.

To make the Seared Sea Scallops, pat the scallops dry on both sides and sprinkle each side with the curry powder. (I prefer not to salt my scallops as I believe they're naturally salty enough, but it's really dependent on your taste.) In a large nonstick skillet over medium-high heat, warm the butter and olive oil until shimmering. You want the skillet to be hot enough that the scallops sizzle upon contact. Add the scallops, in batches if necessary, to avoid overcrowding, and sear on the first side for 2 minutes, then flip and sear another 1½ to 2 minutes until golden-brown on both sides.

Divide the greens among 2 to 3 serving plates and add some mango salsa. Place the scallops on top. Serve with the extra salsa along side.

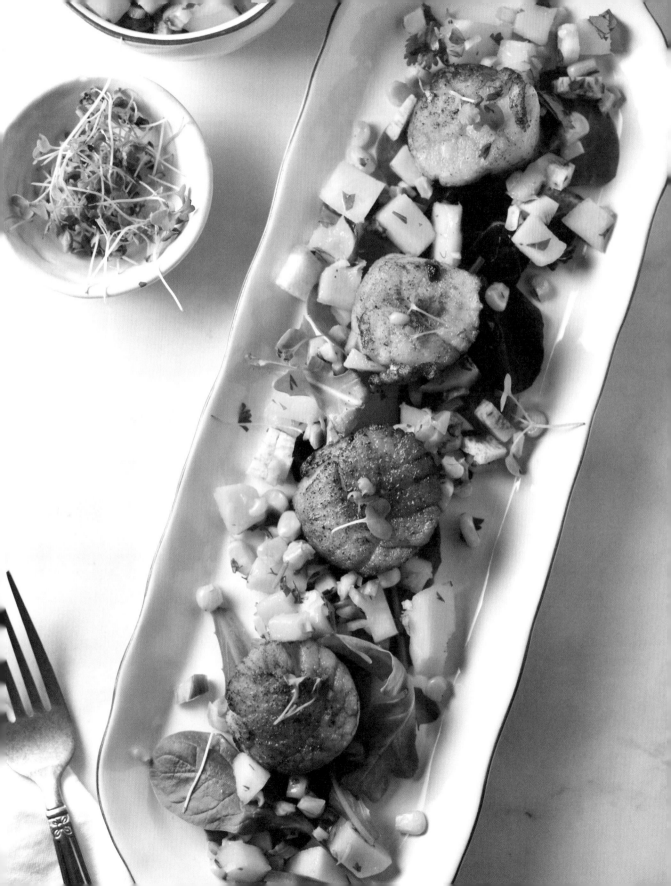

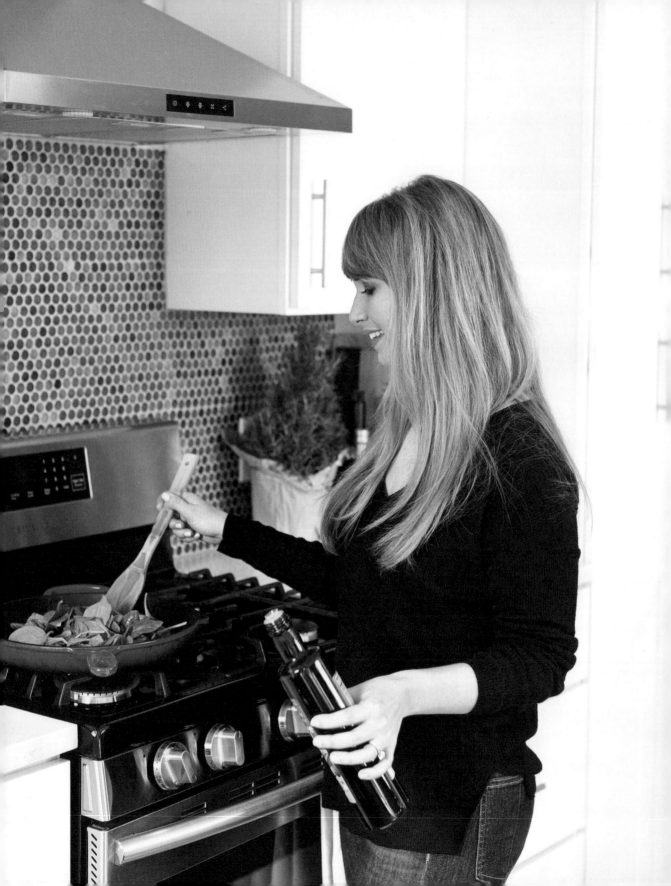

Seriously Good Sides

These recipes are more than just side dishes—some of them could be the star of the whole show. Anyone who is vegetarian and trying to follow a migraine diet will love this chapter, as it contains some of my favorite recipes in the entire book.

The Smoky Sweet Potatoes are the perfect accompaniment for any grilled meat, and we enjoy them weekly with grilled burgers or chicken sandwiches. The Whipped Parsnips, which are nutty and a little sweet, not only pair with rich meals like the Hearty Wine-Free Short Ribs but also with a simple pan-seared salmon. Quick weeknight staples that also pass for date night are the Asparagus with Fresh Dill Vinaigrette and the Garlic Spinach & Tomatoes.

Easily one of my favorite recipes in this whole book, the Mac & Fresh Cheese, made me not miss aged cheeses like Parmesan and sharp cheddar one bit. Even my friends and family can't tell that this is made completely migraine friendly. When I tested this recipe, I brought all my friends over one night for a cooking class. I knew if they could pull it off, even the newest of cooks could definitely recreate this dish for their families. If you have a little more time in the kitchen or are celebrating a special moment, make it. On another cheesy night, the Boursin Scalloped Potatoes are sure to be a hit too.

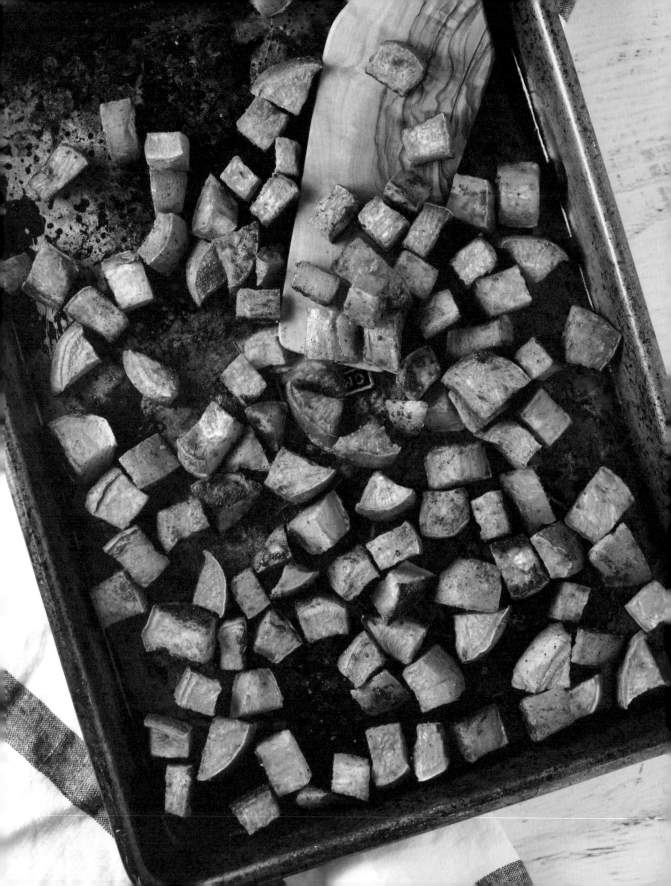

Smoky Sweet Potatoes

MAKES 4 SERVINGS

Just because you are on an elimination diet doesn't mean you have to eliminate flavor—these sweet potatoes are a good example. With a hint of smokiness and spice, these sweet potatoes are a great side for grilled chicken, steak, or burgers. You can also add them to a vegetarian version of the Salsa Verde Chicken Enchiladas (page 137).

1½ pounds sweet potatoes
2 tablespoons olive oil
1 teaspoon smoked paprika
1 teaspoon kosher salt
½ teaspoon garlic powder

Preheat the oven to 425°F and line a large baking sheet with parchment paper.

Scrub the sweet potatoes well under cold running water. Pat the potatoes dry and cut them into ½-inch cubes (there's no need to peel). Transfer cubes to center of the prepared baking sheet and add the olive oil, smoked paprika, salt, and garlic powder. Stir to combine.

Roast until the sweet potatoes are brown and crispy on the outside and tender on the inside, 30 to 35 minutes total, using a spatula to flip the potatoes halfway through. Serve immediately.

Winter Rice Pilaf

MAKES 4 TO 6 SERVINGS

The flavors in this dish are warm and cozy, but I sometimes find myself making it in the middle of summer because it is just that good. Serve along with baked fish or chicken, next to a simple roasted pork tenderloin, or on its own as a hearty vegetarian meal. If you can't find sulfite-free dried cranberries, fresh pomegranate seeds make a great substitute. Just be sure to wait until the end to add them, instead of baking them in the dish.

1 tablespoon olive oil

1 shallot, chopped

1 cup brown rice or rice pilaf blend

⅓ cup dried cranberries (sulfite-free)

1½ teaspoons minced fresh rosemary

1 bay leaf

½ teaspoon kosher salt, plus more to taste

2 cups Vegetable Broth (page 80)

¼ cup pepitas (pumpkin seeds), toasted

Preheat the oven to 400°F.

In an oven-safe medium saucepan, warm the olive oil over medium heat. Add the shallot and sauté until softened, about 2 minutes. Stir in the rice, dried cranberries, rosemary, bay leaf, salt, and broth. Cover with a lid and place in the oven. Bake until the rice has fully absorbed the broth, 35 to 40 minutes.

Discard the bay leaf, stir in the toasted pepitas and salt to taste, and serve.

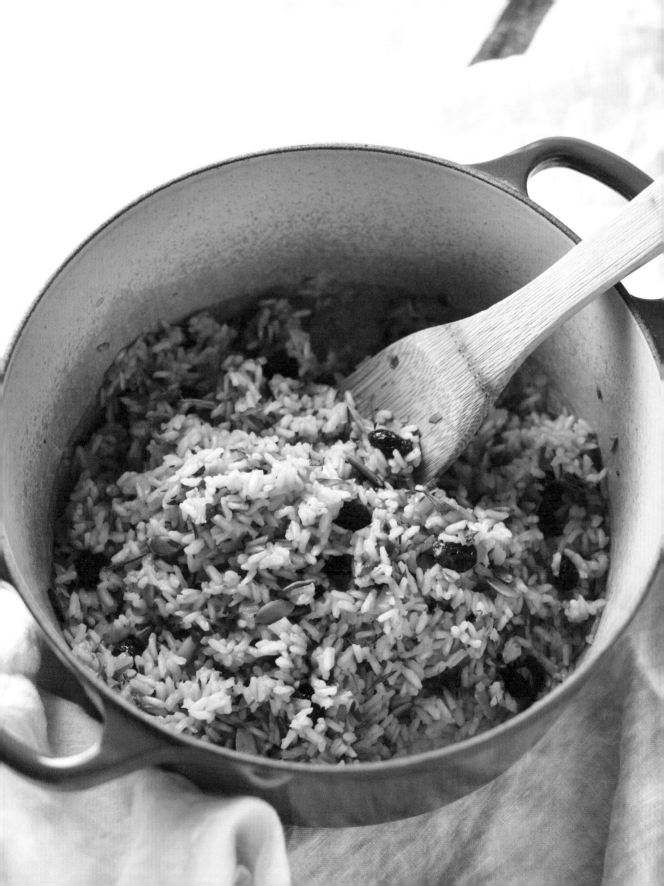

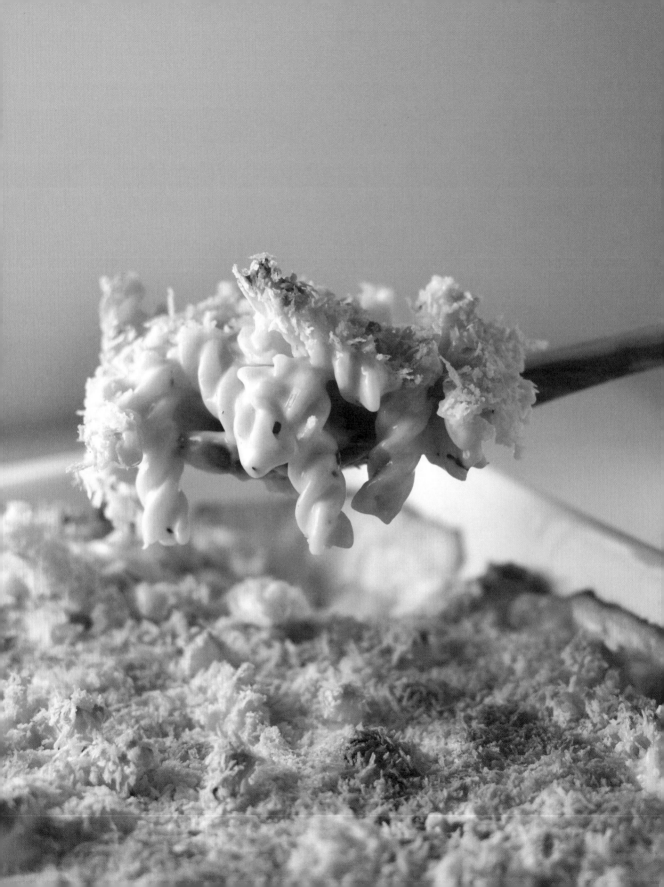

Mac & Fresh Cheese

MAKES 6 SERVINGS

There aren't many recipes out there for mac & cheese that don't contain lots of aged cheese like sharp cheddar and Parmesan. I was afraid that by only using fresh cheeses I would lose a lot of the flavor, but the tasty homemade béchamel (white sauce), thyme, and mustard round everything out. One way I still see my friends with this illness is by inviting them over for meals where I can control my surroundings and what goes into my food. In fact, I tested this recipe by having a little cooking class where I showed my pals how easy it is to roast chicken and make this mac & cheese from scratch. Now this is all my best friend makes for every potluck and holiday dinner she goes to. If my friends can do it, I promise that you can too! For a gluten-free option, use 2 tablespoons brown rice flour and 2 tablespoons tapioca flour, as well as gluten-free panko and pasta.

¾ pound macaroni or other small pasta shape of your choice

2 ¾ cups whole milk

3 tablespoons unsalted butter, plus extra for greasing casserole dish

¼ cup all-purpose flour

½ teaspoon dried thyme

1 teaspoon kosher salt

½ teaspoon dry mustard

¼ teaspoon freshly ground black pepper

2 ¼ cups white American cheese, grated

6 ounces fresh goat cheese (chèvre) (about 1 cup), crumbled

½ cup panko

Bring a large pot of salted water to a boil and pour in the pasta. Cook the pasta for about 4 minutes, or half of what the package time recommends. The pasta should be softened but undercooked. Drain the pasta and rinse under cool water to stop the cooking. Set aside.

Preheat the oven to 375°F and rub a 9-by-13-inch casserole dish with butter. In a small saucepan, warm the milk over medium heat. In a large, deep skillet, melt the 3 tablespoons butter over medium heat, and then whisk in flour until smooth. Allow it to bubble while you continue whisking until the mixture becomes a nice, golden brown color and smells a little nutty. Be careful not to let it go into the dark-brown (burned) territory.

Add the warm milk to the flour-butter mixture about ½ cup at a time, whisking with each addition until smooth. Whisk continuously over medium heat until all the milk has been added and the sauce is thick and smooth, about 10 minutes total. It will be done when it's thick enough to leave a line when you move a spoon through it. Stir in the thyme, salt, dry mustard, and black pepper. Over low heat, add the American cheese one handful at a time, stirring with each addition until fully combined. Then add the goat cheese and stir until smooth. Finally, stir in the cooked pasta. Transfer the mixture to the buttered casserole dish and top with panko.

Bake until browned on top and bubbly, 25 to 30 minutes. Serve warm.

Asparagus with Fresh Dill Vinaigrette

MAKES 4 SERVINGS

My trip to France in 2018 was the second time I had traveled internationally since being diagnosed with VM. I went all out—I had aged cheese and good wine almost every night. There are some moments in life where you just have to take a chance. In Burgundy, there's a Michelin-rated restaurant on almost every corner, so eating adventurously was tough to pass up. I remember craving a salad at one point, and when I mentioned this to my waiter, he laughed and said, "Salad is what the food in Burgundy eats!" There was one meal where we were served blanched asparagus with tons of fresh herbs and chopped hardboiled egg on top. I've rarely branched out of my roasted asparagus routine, but this version was so delicious I knew I had to create my own migraine-safe spin.

1½ pounds fresh asparagus

1 large egg (optional)

2 tablespoons olive oil

2 teaspoons Dijon mustard (wine- and sulfite-free)

1 teaspoon distilled white vinegar

1 small shallot, minced

2 teaspoons roughly chopped fresh dill, plus more for garnish

Kosher salt and freshly ground black pepper

Bring a large pot of salted water to a boil. Prepare an ice bath (a large bowl of water with ice cubes). Trim the thick, woody ends from the asparagus and discard. Rinse spears under cool water. When the water comes to a boil, add the asparagus and cook until crisp-tender, 1½ to 2 minutes. Immediately remove them with tongs and place into the ice bath to stop the cooking. Once cool, dry with paper towels and transfer to a serving platter.

Meanwhile, if you're making a hardboiled egg, bring a small pot of water to a boil. Turn the heat down so the water just simmers, add the shelled egg, and cook for 10 to 12 minutes. Plunge the egg into ice water to stop the cooking. When cool enough to handle, peel and roughly chop the egg. Set aside.

In a small bowl, whisk together the oil, mustard, vinegar, shallot, and dill. Season with salt and pepper to taste, then lightly pour over the asparagus (you may have a small amount of dressing left over). Sprinkle more dill and the egg (if using), over the top. Serve immediately.

> **EASE UP ON VACATION** In his book *Heal Your Headache*, Dr. Buchholz mentions that some patients can get away with eating noncompliant foods on vacation since their migraine threshold is raised by being in a stress-free environment. For those planning a vacation and worrying about how this diet fits in, I highly recommend cutting yourself some slack while still following the diet where you can. There's no need to "start over" after you return, just get strict again and carry on.

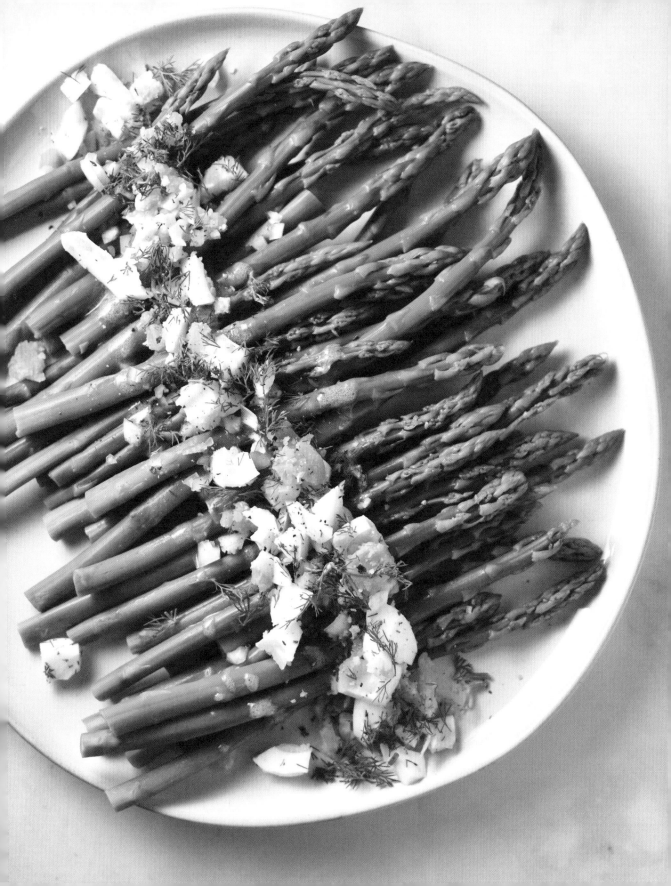

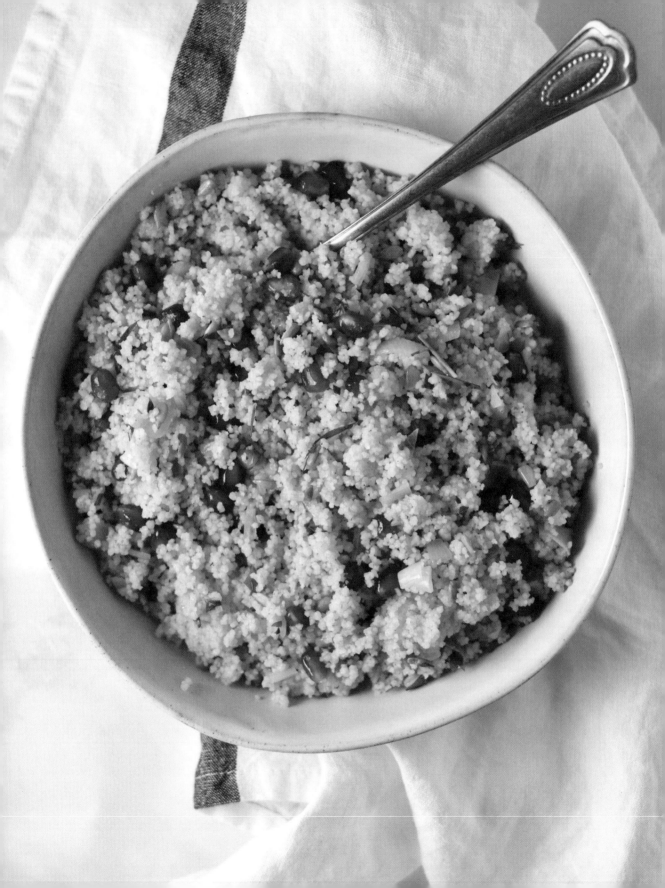

Pomegranate Couscous

MAKES 4 TO 6 SERVINGS

Fresh pomegranate seeds make this a pretty side dish for a potluck party. My favorite way to serve it is alongside the Moroccan Meatballs (page 138) or any simply grilled meat. Make sure that you use regular couscous, which is small and grainy, not the big pearls known as Israeli couscous. There's a big difference in cooking times and liquid amounts between the two!

2 tablespoons unsalted butter

1 shallot, chopped

1½ cups Vegetable Broth (page 80)

¾ cup dried quick-cooking couscous

1 teaspoon paprika

⅓ cup pomegranate seeds

⅓ cup sunflower seeds, toasted

2 tablespoons chopped fresh parsley

Kosher salt and freshly ground black pepper

In a deep skillet with a lid, melt the butter over medium heat. Add the shallot and sauté until softened, 1 to 2 minutes. Add the broth and bring to a boil, then add the couscous, stirring just until combined. Turn off the heat and cover with the lid for 10 minutes—no peeking!

Remove the lid and fluff the couscous with a fork. Stir in the paprika, pomegranate seeds, sunflower seeds, and parsley. Season to taste with salt and pepper, and serve.

Garlic Spinach & Tomatoes

MAKES 2 TO 4 SERVINGS

We all have those dishes that we loved eating out before we started an elimination diet. This is inspired by one of mine, from a little local restaurant that's been a Dallas staple for years. Perhaps I loved it so much because it's drenched in white wine. I did give up wine for a while, but I was eventually able to reintroduce it again—especially organic and biodynamic types. So, don't ever think you have to give up some of your favorite foods forever. It does get better! This dish works well with nearly everything, but I love it with grilled steaks or the Anyone-Can-Cook Roast Chicken. Since this cooks so fast, sometimes I'll place it in a small casserole dish to keep warm in the oven. It holds up well while you finish the rest of the meal.

---

1 tablespoon unsalted butter

1 clove garlic, thinly sliced

½ pint cherry tomatoes, halved

⅓ cup Vegetable Broth (page 80) or Chicken Stock (page 81)

1 (6-ounce) package fresh baby spinach

Kosher salt and black pepper to taste

In a large skillet, melt the butter over medium heat. Add the garlic and sauté until fragrant, 1 to 2 minutes. Add the tomatoes and broth, simmering until the broth is reduced by one-third and the tomatoes are softened, about 4 minutes. Add the spinach and stir until just barely wilted, about 1 minute. Season to taste with salt and pepper, and serve.

SAVVY SUBSTITUTION If you find you are sensitive to tomatoes, just leave them out and increase the amount of spinach you use.

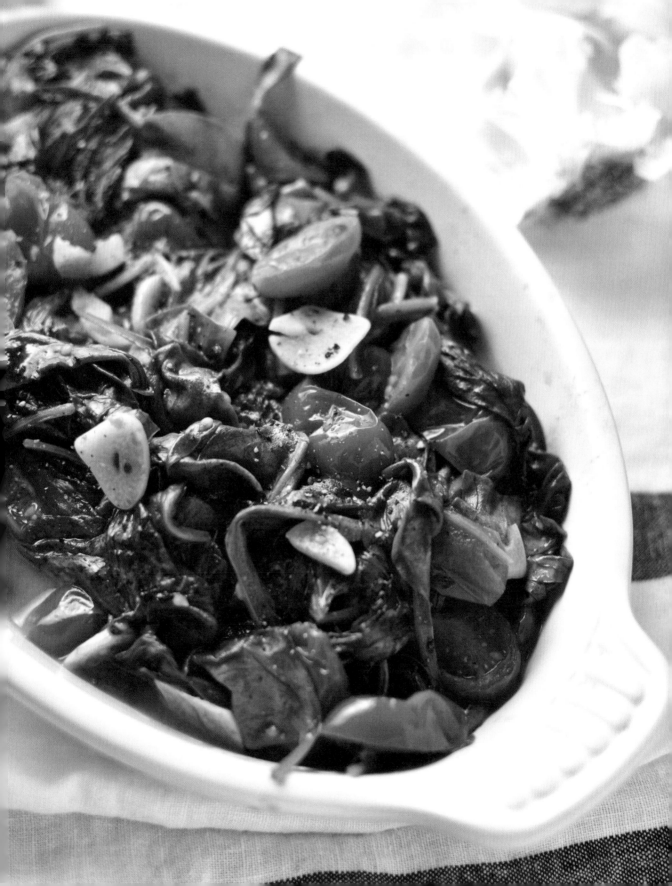

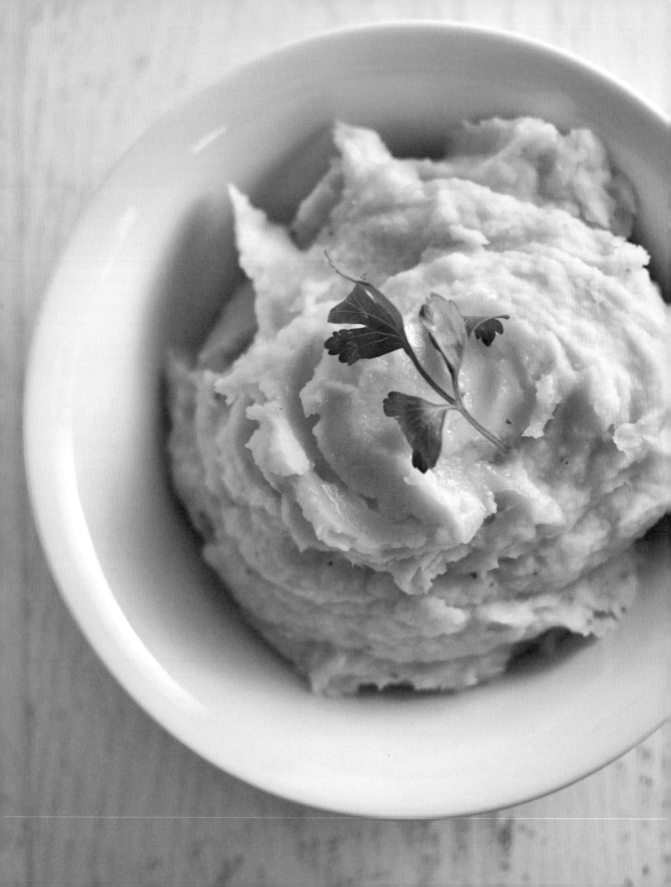

Whipped Parsnips

MAKES 2 TO 4 SERVINGS

You don't see parsnips often in recipes, but they're one of my favorite root vegetables. Similar to carrots but with a cream-colored exterior, they're a little bit sweet. You can cut parsnips into long pieces and roast them as "fries," or you can whip them up into this creamy and glorious side dish. Occasionally, my mother and I can even pass this dish off as "mashed potatoes" to my poor father, who doesn't branch out much in the root vegetable department. These parsnips are wonderful with simply seared fish or the Hearty Wine-Free Short Ribs (page 158).

---

1 pound parsnips, peeled and cut into 2-inch pieces

¼ cup Vegetable Broth (page 80) or Chicken Stock (page 81)

1 tablespoon unsalted butter

½ clove garlic

1 teaspoon kosher salt

Freshly ground black pepper

Bring a small saucepan of water to boil and add the parsnips. Boil until a fork inserted into the parsnips meets no resistance, about 10 minutes. Drain and set aside.

To a large food processor or blender, add the broth, butter, and garlic; pulse until the garlic is chopped. Add the cooked parsnips and salt; pulse until smooth. Season with pepper to taste. Serve hot.

Roasted Curried Cauliflower

MAKES 2 TO 4 SERVINGS

If you're looking for a good way to jazz up your typical roasted cauliflower, then this is the recipe for you. I love to use turmeric in a lot of my cooking because it contains curcumin, an ingredient that has major anti-inflammatory and pain-fighting power. Not only do you get a delicious side dish, but it also might help lessen discomfort on those bad days. This dish is so flavorful that it's best paired with meals that don't have a lot of ingredients—plain burgers, simply seasoned grilled chicken or shrimp, steaks, etc. It can also be served by itself, perhaps with a green salad, as a vegan meal.

---

2 cloves garlic, finely chopped

1½ teaspoons curry powder

1 teaspoon ground turmeric

½ teaspoon ground cumin

3 tablespoons olive oil

1 large head cauliflower,
   cut into large florets

¼ dried cranberries
   (sulfite-free) or fresh
   pomegranate seeds

¼ cup unsalted sunflower
   seeds, toasted

Kosher salt

Chopped fresh parsley
   for garnish (optional)

Preheat oven to 425°F.

In a large bowl, stir together the garlic, curry powder, turmeric, cumin, and olive oil. Add the cauliflower florets and toss until well coated. Pour the coated cauliflower into a single layer onto a baking sheet, leaving some space between the florets. Roast the cauliflower, tossing halfway through, until lightly browned, 20 to 25 minutes. Remove from oven.

Add the dried cranberries or pomegranate seeds and the sunflower seeds to the roasted cauliflower; toss to combine. Taste and add salt, if desired. Garnish with chopped parsley, if desired. Serve warm.

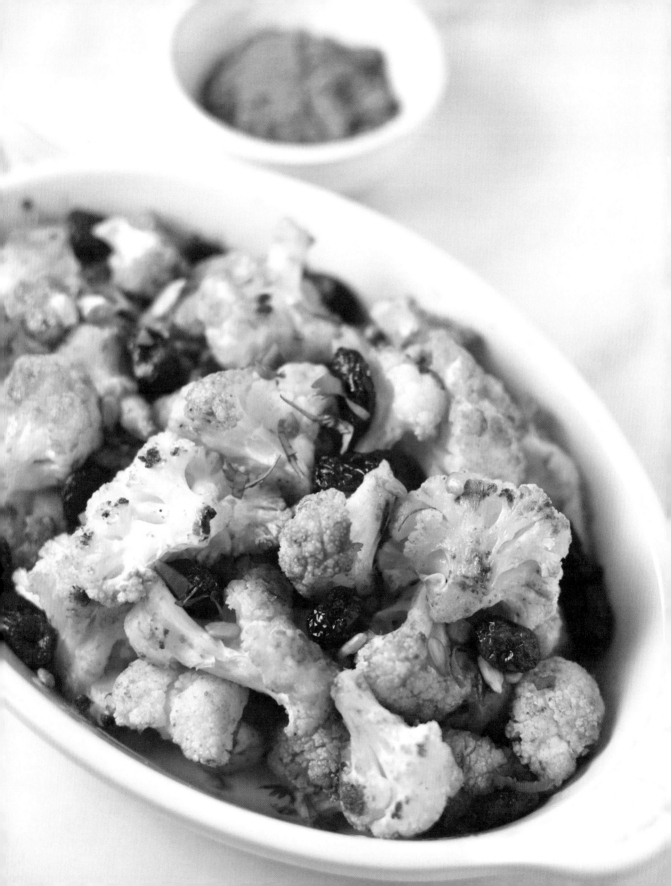

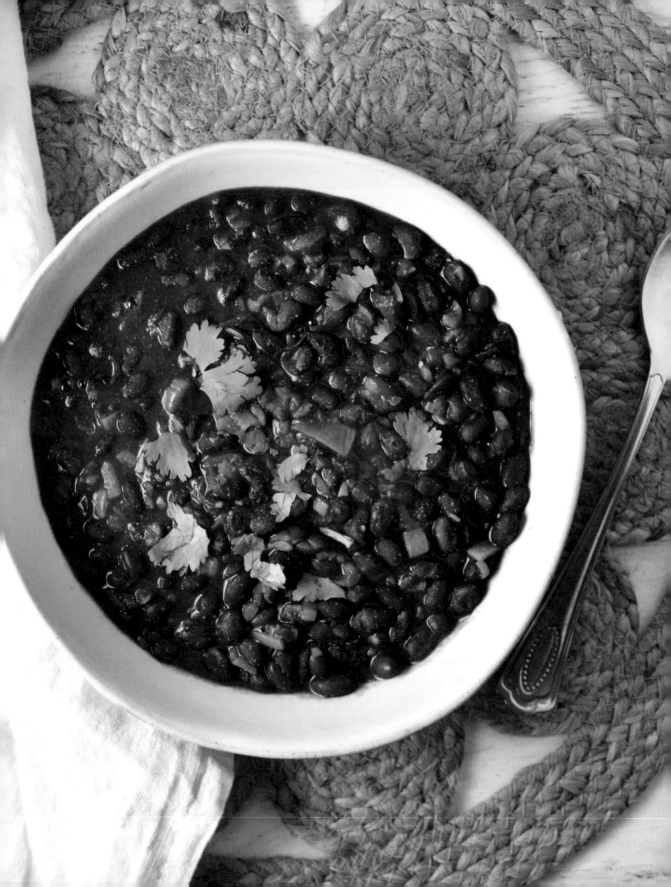

Mexican-Style Black Beans

MAKES 2 TO 4 SERVINGS

There are a few beans out there that should be avoided due to high tyramine content, but black beans are thankfully not one of them. I was never a huge fan of them until I started to incorporate more vegetarian meals into our week, at which point I realized they're incredibly important for both flavor and substance. This version is one of my absolute favorites. It pairs well with the Grilled Chipotle Steak Fajita Bowls (page 157) or with a little bit of Oaxaca or American cheese in a simple quesadilla. When shopping, look for low-sodium beans packed in water.

1 (15.5 ounce) can low-sodium black beans packed in water, not drained

1 small shallot, minced

¼ cup Vegetable Broth (page 80)

2 teaspoons distilled white vinegar

1 teaspoon garlic powder

½ teaspoon chipotle chile powder

½ teaspoon ground cumin

¼ teaspoon dried oregano

1 bay leaf

Kosher salt to taste

Roughly chopped fresh cilantro for garnish (optional)

In a small saucepan, stir together the beans and their liquid, shallot, broth, vinegar, garlic powder, chipotle powder, cumin, oregano, and bay leaf. Bring to a simmer over medium-low heat. Cook until warmed through, stirring often, 10 to 15 minutes. Season to taste with salt. Garnish with chopped cilantro, if desired, and serve warm.

> **EATING BEANS ON HYH** Beans can be confusing on the HYH eating plan, especially since many low-tyramine migraine diets have different lists. This is where following one single elimination list comes in handy. Fava beans, lima beans, navy beans, and broad beans are the most tyramine rich, so it's recommended to avoid those in the elimination stage.

Boursin Scalloped Potatoes

MAKES 4 TO 6 SERVINGS

Ah, scalloped potatoes. Typically covered in tons of butter, cheese, and cream, it's the stuff my Christmas dinner dreams are made of. I found that Boursin brand Garlic & Fine Herbs cheese makes it creamy without heavy cream and packs a ton of flavor without resorting to unfriendly aged cheeses. Boursin is essentially a glorified (as it should be) cream cheese that you can find at most grocery stores. If you're like me, it will become your new best friend throughout your first few months on a migraine diet. These potatoes rarely make it to the dinner table without me taking out a corner to "taste test."

Olive oil for greasing dish

2 pounds Yukon Gold potatoes, unpeeled

2 tablespoons unsalted butter

2 medium shallots, chopped

2 cloves garlic, minced

1 tablespoon all-purpose flour

1 cup whole milk

½ cup Vegetable Broth (page 80) or Chicken Stock (page 81)

1 teaspoon kosher salt

¼ teaspoon dried thyme

Freshly ground black pepper

1 (5.2-ounce) package Boursin Garlic & Fine Herbs Cheese

Chopped fresh parsley for garnish (optional)

Preheat the oven to 400°F. Grease a 9-by-13-inch baking dish with a little olive oil. Slice the potatoes ¼-inch thick. Arrange one layer of potato slices in the bottom of the dish, reserving the remaining slices.

In a medium saucepan, melt the butter over medium heat. Add the shallots and garlic. Sauté until shallots are translucent and soft but not brown, about 2 minutes. Add the flour and stir to combine. Slowly whisk in the milk followed by the broth until everything is smooth. Stir in salt, thyme, and black pepper to taste. Bring the mixture to a simmer over medium heat and cook until thickened, about 5 minutes. Remove from the heat and whisk in the Boursin until smooth and creamy.

Spoon a few tablespoons of the sauce over the first layer of potatoes in the dish, smoothing out over the top. Then add another layer of potatoes, which can slightly overlap, repeating with more sauce on top. If you have more potatoes left over, you can continue to layer them, just save enough sauce to pour on top.

Cover the baking dish with foil and bake for 30 minutes. Remove the foil and bake uncovered until golden brown and bubbling, another 20 minutes. Garnish with parsley, if desired, and serve.

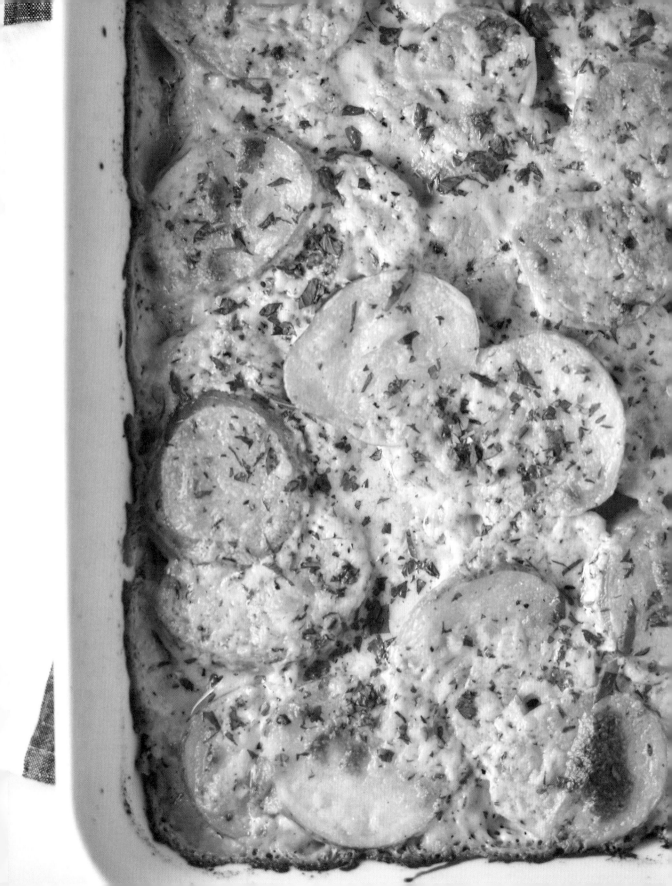

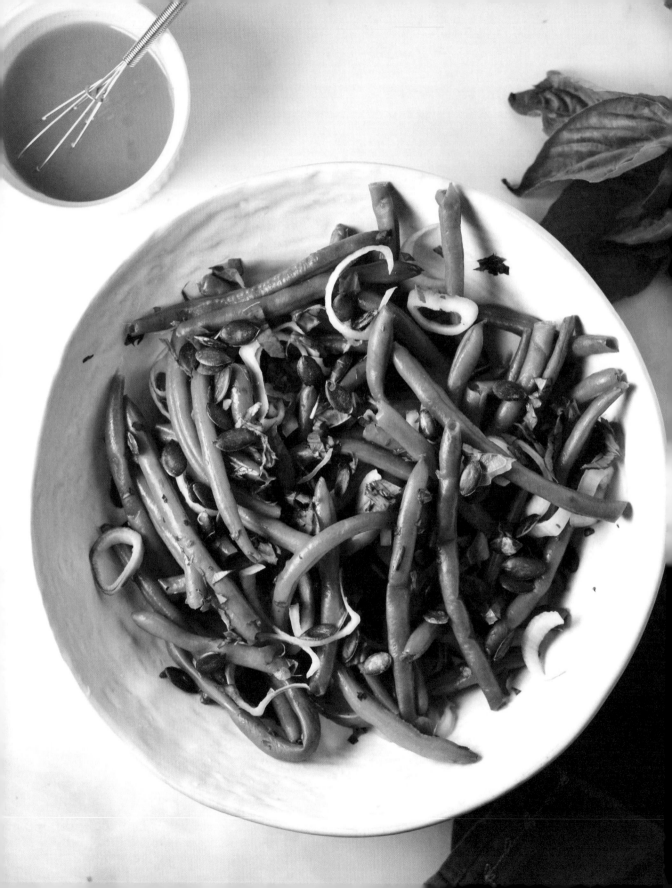

Basil Green Bean Salad

MAKES 4 SERVINGS

Having salads with lettuce night after night can get monotonous, and this herbed salad is the perfect way to mix it up. This recipe uses a technique called parboiling, or blanching, which partially cooks vegetables but without them getting too soft. This method makes the green beans bright and vibrant while maintaining crunch. It's really important to err on the side of less time when boiling these, as mushy green beans are the last thing you want in this salad. If you don't plan to serve this immediately, just keep the dressing separate from the green beans and chill everything until you're ready to dish up some green goodness.

---

1 pound green beans, ends trimmed

¼ cup olive oil

1½ tablespoons distilled white vinegar

1 teaspoon whole-grain mustard (wine- and sulfite-free)

1–2 shallots, thinly sliced

3 tablespoons chopped fresh basil

¼ cup pepitas (pumpkin seeds), toasted

Bring a large saucepan of salted water to a boil. Prepare a large bowl with ice water. When the water comes to a boil, add the trimmed green beans. Cook for exactly 1 minute and 30 seconds, or until crisp-tender, then drain through a colander. Immediately transfer the beans to the ice bath to stop the cooking. Drain and pat dry.

In a small bowl, combine the olive oil, vinegar, and mustard, whisking until smooth. Stir in the shallots.

In a large bowl, toss the dried green beans with the basil and pepitas. Using a slotted spoon, transfer shallots from dressing to the green bean mixture; toss again. Add remaining dressing to taste, and serve.

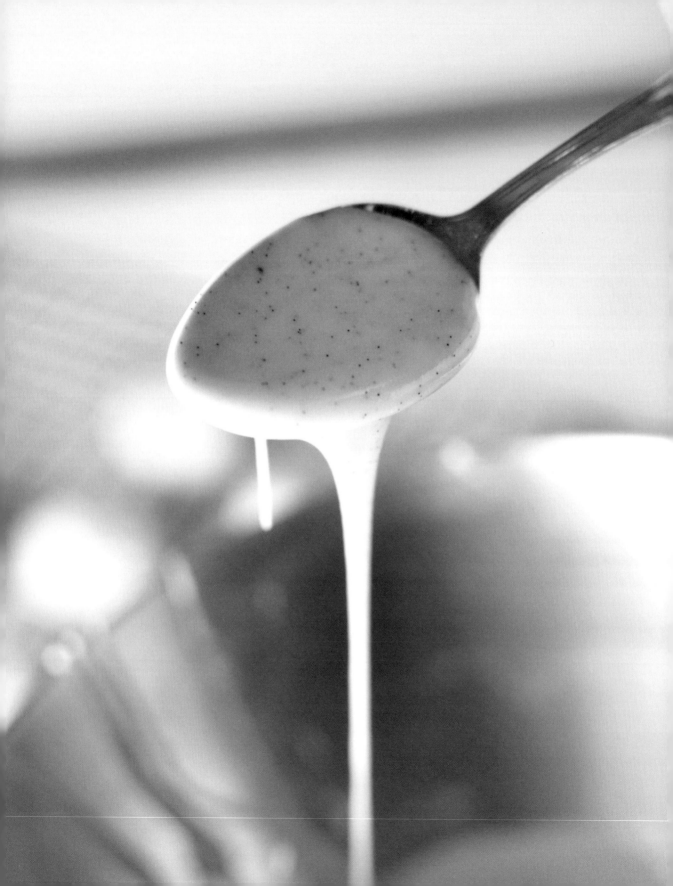

Sweet Treats

An expert baker I am not. Perhaps one day I'll get there if I watch enough *Great British Baking Show*, but I'm way too impatient for the measuring baking requires. Most of the time I eyeball my teaspoons and just throw random spices together. With baking, you really can't do that. So, I keep my baking simple, and the first few recipes in this chapter reflect my baking style.

The next section of recipes comes from my friend Jennifer Bragdon, a.k.a. "The Dizzy Baker." You'll learn more about her on page 206. Her recipes are a little more ambitious but still straightforward and easy to follow.

As you are considering all the tempting treats in this chapter, it's important to note that excessive amounts of sugar can potentially be a migraine trigger. When you eat simple carbohydrates, your blood sugar can rise. In turn, your body produces extra insulin, which causes your blood sugar to drop. Large increases and drops in blood sugar can lead to migraine attacks. My tip for consuming sugar when you live with a migraine disorder is to make sure you're consuming sweet treats with a little bit of protein and fiber. Doing so will help regulate your blood sugar levels so there's not a massive rise and fall. Like most things in life, everything in moderation works best.

I like to keep my cookies in the freezer so I'm not tempted to eat one every day, but they are still there on those days you just need a dang cookie! Just be aware of what you're eating and don't binge a bunch of desserts just because they're "allowed" on this diet.

A super-quick sweet treat is head-friendly vanilla ice cream topped with fruit. I love to sauté a few pears or apples with cinnamon and a tiny bit of butter. When searching for a good vanilla ice cream, look for as few ingredients as possible on the label: milk, eggs, cream, vanilla. Häagen-Dazs makes a stellar one.

Snickerdoodle Cookie Dough Bites

MAKES ABOUT 28 1½-INCH BALLS

If you're anything like me, the best part of baking cookies when you were growing up (or any day, let's be honest) was licking the batter spoon. Finally, here's a cookie dough that you can eat without your mom yelling that you'll get salmonella poisoning! These gluten-free treats are perfect for those times when you're looking for a tiny indulgence.

1¼ cups certified gluten-free
   oat flour
¼ cup white cane sugar
¼ cup packed light brown sugar
2 teaspoons ground cinnamon
¼ teaspoon kosher salt
½ cup unsalted butter,
   at room temperature
2 teaspoons vanilla extract
2–4 tablespoons milk of choice
1¼ cups white chocolate chips

In a large bowl, whisk together the oat flour, white and brown sugars, cinnamon, and salt. Add the softened butter and work it into the flour mixture with a wooden spoon until fully combined. Add vanilla and 2 tablespoons milk. Stir until the dough comes together. Add more milk as needed to form a moist ball of dough.

Line a baking sheet with parchment paper. Using your hands, form the dough into 1½-inch balls and place on the prepared sheet. Freeze until the balls are firm, at least 2 hours.

In a microwave-safe medium bowl, warm the white chocolate chips in the microwave on high power in 30-second increments, stirring with a spoon in between, until fully melted.

Dip each ball in the white chocolate and return to the parchment-lined baking sheet. Allow the coated balls to cool and harden on the counter for a few minutes, then transfer to the freezer for at least 1 hour to completely harden before serving. Store the balls in the freezer in a locking plastic bag until you're ready to eat. The chocolate tends to soften if you leave them at room temperature for a while.

Notes: See Nutty Pancakes (page 65) for tips on making your own oat flour. To substitute all-purpose flour, bake the flour on a baking sheet at 350°F for 5 minutes to decrease the chance of foodborne illness.

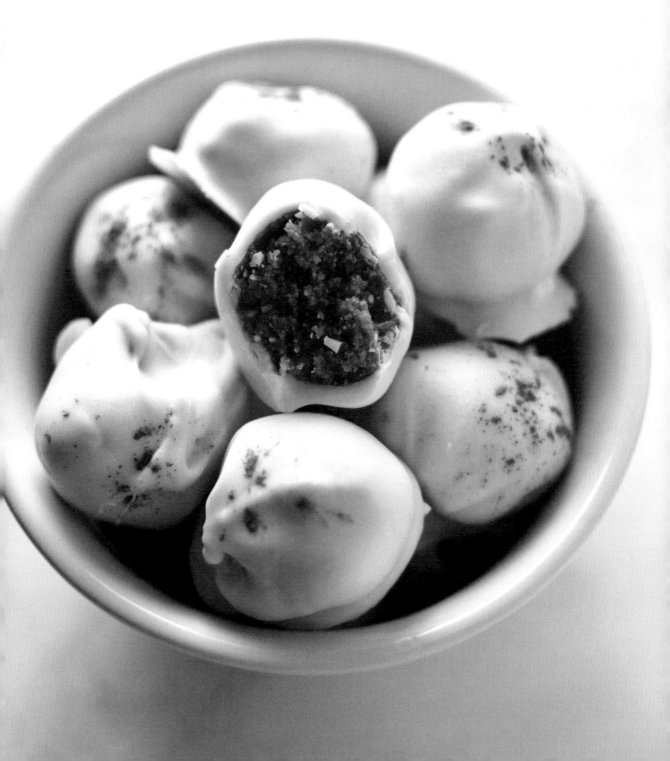

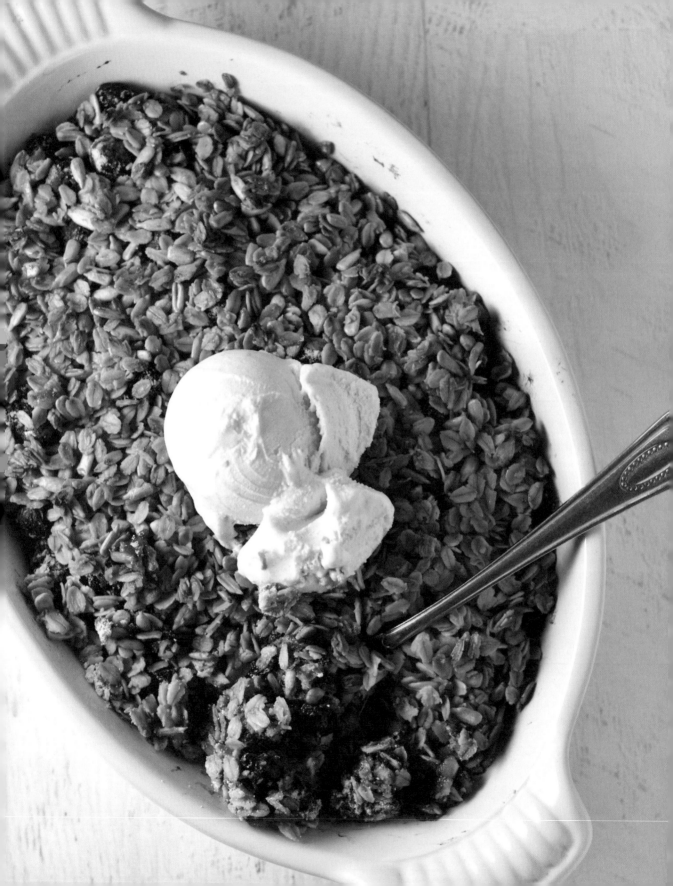

Black & Blue Sunflower Seed Crumble

MAKES 4 TO 6 SERVINGS

Crumbles are some of the easiest summer desserts you can make. You just dump some fresh fruit in a baking dish, cover with oats, toss into the oven, and call it a day. If I'm ever searching for a last-minute dessert idea, it usually falls into this category. The best thing about crumbles is you can assemble everything early in the day and then just bake it right before serving. If you really want to do it right, add a scoop of head-friendly vanilla ice cream (like Häagen-Dazs or McConnell's) on top while it's warm. If you're gluten free, use cornstarch and certified gluten-free oats and oat flour. If you're dairy free, use coconut oil in place of the butter.

Butter or coconut oil
for greasing dish

BERRY FILLING

3 cups fresh blueberries

1 cup fresh blackberries

1½ tablespoons all-purpose
flour or cornstarch

¼ teaspoon ground cinnamon

1 teaspoon vanilla extract

CRUMBLE TOPPING

1¼ cups rolled oats (certified
gluten-free, if desired)

⅓ cup raw sunflower seeds

¼ cup oat flour (certified
gluten-free, if desired)

¼ cup honey

¼ cup unsalted butter or
coconut oil, melted

¼ teaspoon kosher salt

Vanilla ice cream (optional)

Preheat the oven to 350°F with a rack in the center. Grease an 11-inch gratin dish with a little butter. You can also use a 10-inch round or 9-inch square baking pan.

To make the Berry Filling, in a large bowl, stir together the blueberries, blackberries, flour, cinnamon, and vanilla. Transfer the mixture to the prepared dish and spread it out in a single layer. Reserve the large bowl.

To make the Crumble Topping, in the now-empty large bowl, stir together the oats, sunflower seeds, oat flour, honey, melted butter, and salt until crumbly and evenly mixed. Sprinkle on top of the fruit mixture.

Bake until golden brown, 55 to 60 minutes. Cool on a wire rack for about 10 minutes, then dish out into shallow bowls. Top with vanilla ice cream, if desired, and serve warm.

Chewy Ginger Cookies

MAKES 25 COOKIES

This recipe was inspired by one that has been in my mom's family for years. The unfortunate part was my grandma uses butter-flavored shortening in her recipe, which is not an option on this diet. Fake butter flavor? Definitely an MSG red flag! I thought I could just substitute real butter in its place, but the first time I made them they spread out into giant, flat cookies. (Not a total fail—I crushed them up and put them on top of ice cream.) Needless to say, it took a few tries to get this recipe perfect. The most important part is to chill the dough, which will help prevent it from spreading.

---

2 cups all-purpose flour
1 teaspoon ground ginger
1 teaspoon ground cloves
1 teaspoon ground cinnamon
¼ teaspoon table salt
1 teaspoon baking soda
10 tablespoons unsalted butter, at room temperature
¾ cup white cane sugar
¼ cup unsulfured molasses
1 large egg

In a medium bowl, whisk together the flour, ginger, cloves, cinnamon, salt, and baking soda. In a large bowl, cream together the butter and sugar using an electric mixer. Add the molasses and egg. Continue mixing until smooth. Slowly add the flour mixture to the butter and sugar mixture, roughly ¼ cup at a time, and use a wooden spoon to stir until fully combined. Cover the bowl and refrigerate for at least 1 hour.

Preheat oven to 350°F. Line 2 baking sheets with parchment paper or silicone baking mats.

Using your hands, roll the dough into 1½-inch balls and place them on the sheets, spacing at least 2 inches apart. Bake until the cookies are set around the edges, about 13 minutes. Transfer cookies to a wire rack and cool to room temperature before serving.

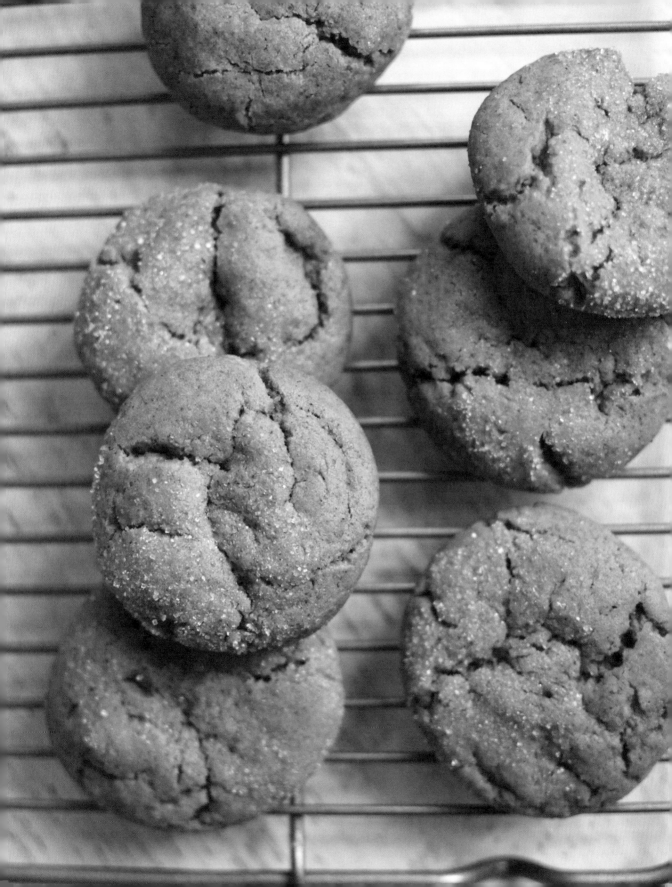

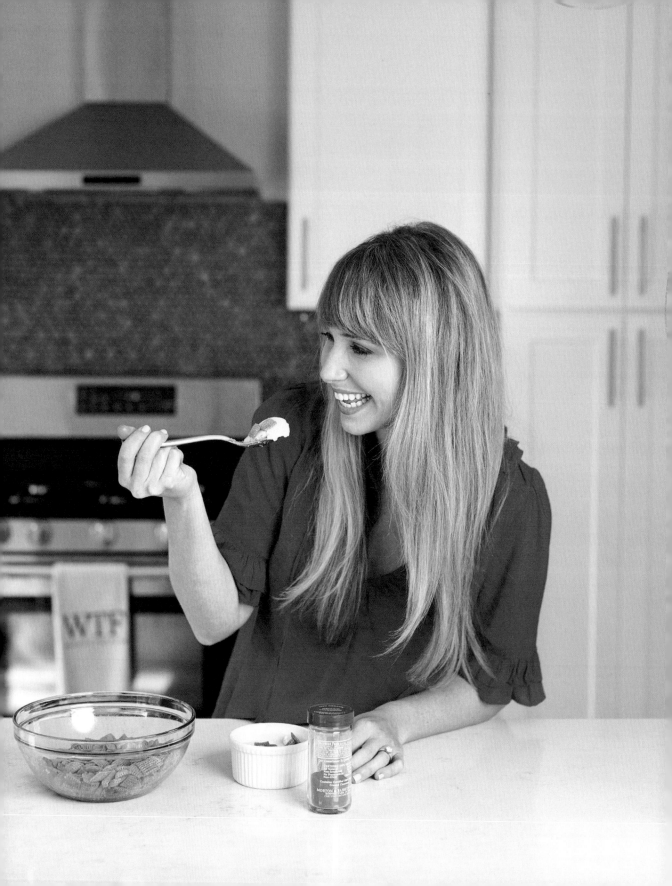

Saturday Morning Cartoon Pudding

MAKES 4 SERVINGS

The boring name for this would be "White Chocolate Pudding with Cinnamon Chex," but I couldn't help but think of cereal and milk while creating this recipe. It brought me back to those days when I used to eat super-sugary cinnamon cereal (Saturdays only) and watch hours of cartoons. The whole thing takes about 15 minutes to come together, and the rest of the time is for chilling. Be careful with the Cinnamon Chex—it's addictive.

WHITE CHOCOLATE PUDDING

3 tablespoons cornstarch

¼ teaspoon kosher salt

2 cups whole milk

½ cup white chocolate chips

1½ teaspoons vanilla extract

CINNAMON CHEX

1 cup rice or corn Chex cereal

1 tablespoon unsalted butter, melted

1 tablespoon white cane sugar

½ teaspoon ground cinnamon

To make the White Chocolate Pudding, in a small saucepan, mix together the cornstarch and salt. Turn the heat to medium-low and whisk in the milk a little bit at a time until smooth. Turn the heat up to medium and bring the mixture to a strong simmer. Simmer, whisking continuously, until slightly thickened, about 5 minutes. Reduce the heat to low and whisk for another 2 minutes. (Be careful not to let the mixture simmer for too long or it will affect the texture.) Add the white chocolate chips, which should melt fairly quickly, and vanilla. Whisk until smooth. Remove from the heat and spoon into 4 individual ½-cup ramekins, dividing evenly. Cover with plastic wrap directly on top of the pudding and refrigerate until set, 1 to 2 hours.

To make the Cinnamon Chex, while the pudding is chilling, stir together the Chex, melted butter, and sugar in a medium microwave-safe bowl. Microwave on high power for 30 seconds, stir, and then microwave for another 30 seconds. Stir in the cinnamon while the mixture is warm. Cool at room temperature, uncovered, until crispy.

Top the chilled puddings with the Cinnamon Chex and serve.

Gooey White Chocolate Blondies

MAKES 12 BLONDIES

I missed chocolate so much during the elimination phase of the HYH diet. My dreams were full of super fudgy, dark chocolate brownies that were jumping into a big bowl of red wine. That's when I got the idea to do a blondie, but my goal was to make one that had a gooey brownie-like texture. Eventually I was able to reintroduce chocolate in moderation, but I still love this recipe. Some white chocolate brands are sweeter than others. For this recipe I use Callebaut, which tends to be a little less sweet. Be sure to give your chocolate a taste test before proceeding with the recipe (I know, so difficult) to see if you should cut back on the added ½ cup of white chocolate pieces.

1½ cups good-quality white chocolate chips or very small pieces cut from a bar (about 12 ounces), divided

½ cup unsalted butter, cut into ½-inch pieces

½ cup white cane sugar

2 extra-large eggs, lightly beaten

1½ teaspoons vanilla extract

½ teaspoon kosher salt

1¼ cups all-purpose flour or gluten-free all-purpose flour (avoid xanthan gum if you're sensitive)

Preheat the oven to 350°F. Line an 8-inch square baking pan with a parchment paper overhang.

In a double boiler or a thick, heatproof mixing bowl set over a pan of simmering water, heat 1 cup of the white chocolate chips and the butter, stirring continuously with a whisk until melted, thick, and glossy. (You want to watch this carefully, so they blend together and do not separate.) Remove from the heat. Add the sugar and whisk to combine. Add the eggs, vanilla, and salt; whisk to combine. Add the flour in ¼-cup increments, using a rubber spatula to fold the batter carefully after each addition until just combined. Finally, stir in the remaining ½ cup of the white chocolate chips. Do not overmix.

Transfer batter to the prepared baking pan. Bake until the blondies are slightly browned on top and a toothpick inserted into the center comes out mostly clean, with a few moist crumbs attached, 28 to 30 minutes. Cool in the pan at least 15 minutes. Using parchment overhang, transfer blondies to a cutting board. Cut into 12 squares and serve.

NOT REALLY CHOCOLATE White chocolate is made from the fat that's been extracted from the cocoa beans rather than from actual cocoa beans, which is what makes it tolerable for migraine sufferers. Soy lecithin is common in white chocolate, and while soy is on the avoid list, this is one ingredient you don't necessarily have to worry about. If you can't tolerate soy at all, don't fret. Many white chocolate brands use sunflower lecithin instead.

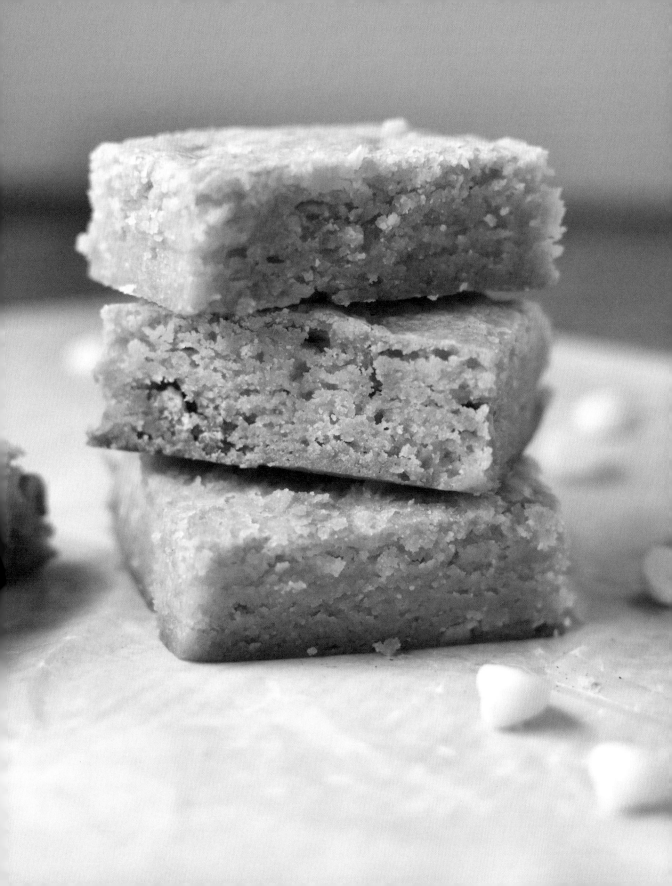

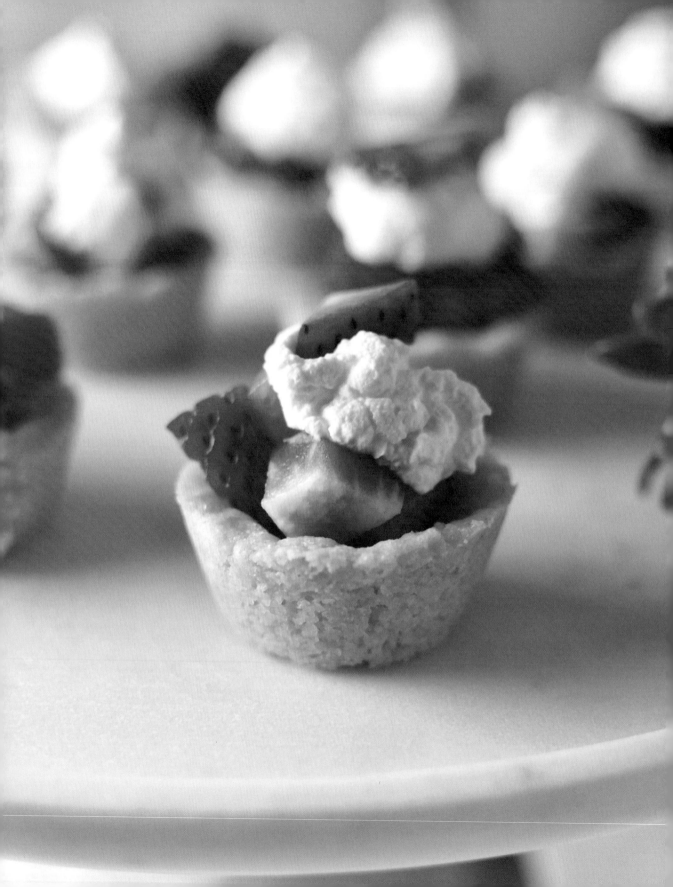

Mini Strawberry Shortcake Cups

MAKES 24 MINI MUFFIN CUPS

These little cups taste like shortbread and are filled with delicious, fresh strawberries and homemade whipped cream. Since the cups freeze easily, they make a great dinner-party dessert. All you have to do is pull them out of the freezer about an hour before you plan to serve them and make the whipped cream at the last minute. I've substituted blueberries for strawberries before, and it's delicious either way. I don't add sugar to my whipped cream here because I think the cups and berries provide the perfect level of sweetness.

COOKIE CUPS

7 tablespoons unsalted butter, at room temperature

1¼ cups all-purpose flour

½ teaspoon baking powder

¼ teaspoon table salt

⅓ cup white cane sugar

1 large egg

1 teaspoon vanilla extract

SHORTCAKE TOPPING

½ cup heavy cream (carrageenan-free), chilled

8 ounces fresh strawberries, chopped

For the Cookie Cups, preheat the oven to 350°F. Grease a 24-cup mini muffin pan with 1 tablespoon of the softened butter, dividing equally.

In a small bowl, whisk together the flour, baking powder, and salt. In a medium bowl, cream together the remaining 6 tablespoons of the softened butter and the sugar using an electric mixer. Add the egg and vanilla, mixing until just combined. Add the flour mixture to the butter mixture a little bit at a time, beating until well mixed. Refrigerate the dough for about 20 minutes.

Form the chilled dough into 24 balls about 1 inch in diameter and place into each muffin cup. Using your thumb, make an indention in each ball, forming a little cup. Poke the tines of a fork into the bottom of each cup to create tiny holes. Bake the cups until lightly browned, 12 to 15 minutes. If the cups are raised in the middle, gently press down on the warm dough with your thumb to create a bigger indention for the strawberries. Cool in the pan for about 5 minutes, then transfer to a wire rack to cool completely.

When you're ready to serve, make the Shortcake Topping: Whip the heavy cream with an electric mixer at medium-high speed until firm peaks form, 3 to 4 minutes. Fill each cup with strawberry pieces and top with the fresh whipped cream. Serve immediately.

Introducing The Dizzy Baker

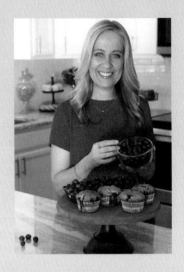

Migraine support groups can be a double-edged sword when you're not feeling well, but there is so much hope and inspiration tucked away in them. It was in one of these support groups, called Migraine Strong, that I first met Alicia. We both got sick with chronic vestibular migraine (VM) around the same time, and I found myself gravitating toward people who were making small gains, allowing opportunities for education rather than expressing the fear and uncertainty that comes with this diagnosis. We chatted here and there, helping each other navigate toward our recovery. As an administrator for Migraine Strong, our team was so excited to see Alicia create a resource for people on one of the migraine diets we support on her site, TheDizzyCook.com. Since I occasionally posted head-safe baking recipes (like my famous blueberry muffins on page 50!) for our group, I teased that I couldn't wait to be a guest baker on Alicia's site. To my surprise, she welcomed me with open arms, and The Dizzy Baker was officially born.

Once a month, I share my journey with VM, the tips and tricks I've learned, plus a new recipe. Together, Alicia and I help others out of daily dizziness, and behind the scenes we help each other through our toughest days. Although we have never met in person, we consider each other to be close friends, connected through adversity. The experience of navigating chronic migraine is hard, but it has brought me many gifts, including friendship. Sometimes I actually feel grateful for going through it.

I hope my recipes inspire you to make baking a part of your treatment plan. Baking is not just about eating. It's a great way to change your focus when you are experiencing difficult symptoms. Research tells us creative activities take up so much room in your brain that it's difficult to feel pain while you're engaging in them. I've experienced this firsthand.

Baking requires slow, focused concentration, allowing you to be fully present in the moment. This leads to mindfulness that doesn't allow time for negative thoughts to creep in. In addition to its physical health benefits, baking strengthens mental health because it can be an expression of love. Giving something you created to another person fosters your own feelings of accomplishment and purpose. It's a way to contribute joy to your family when you find engaging in other tasks to be difficult. Not to mention, it's tough to feel despair in a house that smells like cookies! If you're having a bad day, seeing your beautiful creations will remind you of the sweet things in life. And that, my friends, is the icing on the cake! —Jennifer Bragdon

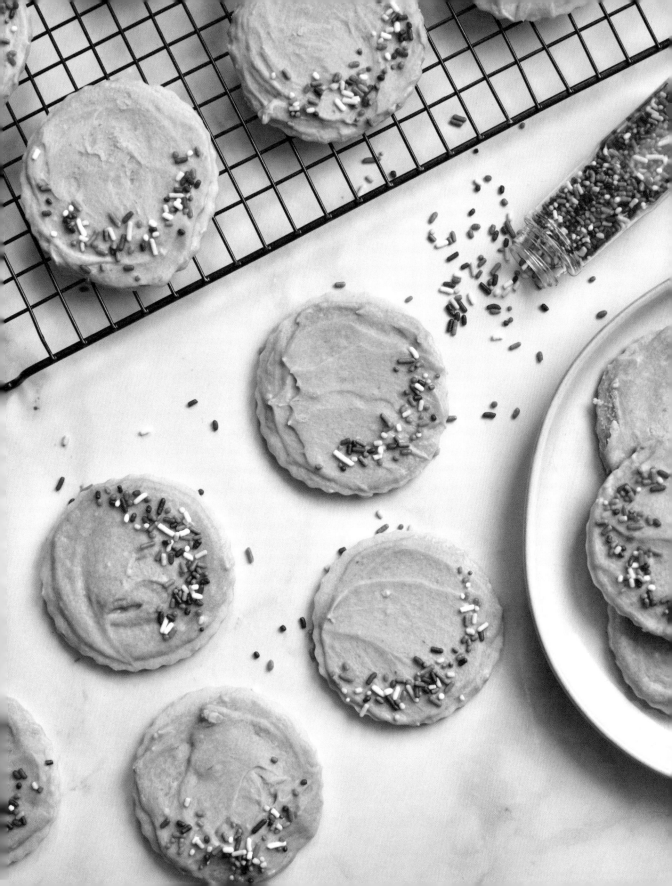

Cream Cheese Sugar Cookies with Cherry Frosting

RECIPE BY THE DIZZY BAKER • MAKES ABOUT 36 3-INCH COOKIES

Sugar cookies are my all-time favorite. Topped with frosting and cut into festive shapes, there is no other cookie that's this fun to eat. I created this clean version by cutting out the food coloring and using real fruit to color the frosting. The result is better than the version from my childhood. Sometimes I can hardly believe that I haven't baked like this all along! Make sure you use block cream cheese and not a spreadable brand, like Arla, or the cookies and frosting will not have the correct texture. —JB

CREAM CHEESE SUGAR COOKIES

3 cups all-purpose flour

1½ teaspoons baking powder

½ teaspoon table salt

1 cup unsalted butter, at room temperature

4 ounces cream cheese (carrageenan-free), at room temperature

¾ cups white cane sugar

1 large egg, at room temperature

2 teaspoons vanilla extract

To make the Cream Cheese Sugar Cookies, in a medium bowl, whisk together the flour, baking powder, and salt until blended. In a large bowl, combine the butter and cream cheese using an electric mixer on high speed. Beat until smooth and creamy, about 2 minutes. Add sugar and beat on medium-high speed until fluffy and light in color. Add the egg and vanilla, beating until well blended, about 1 minute. Slowly add the flour mixture to the butter mixture; beat on low speed until just combined. The dough will be very soft and creamy.

Lightly flour your work surface, rolling pin, and hands. Divide the dough into 2 equal portions. Roll out each portion onto a piece of wax paper or a silicone baking mat to about ¼-inch thickness. The rolled-out dough can be any shape, as long as it is evenly ¼-inch thick. Transfer the rolled-out dough on the wax paper to a baking sheet and cover it with another sheet of wax paper. Roll out the second portion of dough in the same manner and stack it on top of the first piece of dough on the baking sheet. Cover the top with a sheet of wax paper. Refrigerate the rolled-out and stacked dough for at least 2 hours.

When you're ready to bake, preheat the oven to 350°F. Line 2 large baking sheets with parchment paper or silicone baking mats. Remove one of the dough pieces from the refrigerator and peel off the top layer of wax paper. Using a 3-inch-round cookie cutter, cut the dough into as many rounds as possible. Transfer the dough rounds to the

CHERRY FROSTING

1 cup frozen pitted
  dark cherries

1 cup unsalted butter,
  at room temperature

4 ounces cream cheese
  (carrageenan-free),
  at room temperature

Pinch of table salt

1 teaspoon vanilla extract

2 cups powdered sugar,
  plus more if needed

Heavy cream (carrageenan-
  free) or milk, if needed

Sprinkles for decorating
  (optional)

prepared baking sheets, spacing 1-inch apart. Re-roll the remaining dough and continue cutting until all the dough is used. Repeat the cutting process with the second piece of dough.

Bake until the cookies are lightly browned around the edges, 11 to 12 minutes. Allow the cookies to cool on the baking sheet for 5 minutes, then transfer them to a wire rack to cool completely before you begin decorating. The frosting will spread unevenly if the cookies are too warm.

To make the Cherry Frosting, add the frozen cherries to a small saucepan and simmer on medium-low heat until the cherries are soft, and the liquid has reduced, about 15 minutes. Carefully pour the cherries into a food processor or blender and puree until smooth. Set aside to cool.

In a medium mixing bowl, beat the butter with an electric mixer until it's light and fluffy, about 2 to 4 minutes, but take your time with this. The butter will look yellow in the beginning and will turn to more of a light cream color when it's been sufficiently whipped. Add the cream cheese, pinch of salt, and vanilla. Mix until combined, then mix in a ¼ cup of the cherry puree. Slowly mix in the powdered sugar. The frosting should look light and creamy. If the consistency is too thin, add more powdered sugar. If it's too thick, add a bit of cream or milk. If the color of the frosting isn't to your liking, add additional cherry puree. (Freeze any leftover cherry puree for future baking.)

Once the cookies are completely cool, spread on the frosting. Return the frosted cookies to the baking sheets and add sprinkles if you wish. Refrigerate for at least 1 hour to firm the frosting before serving. Store the frosted cookies in an airtight container in the refrigerator.

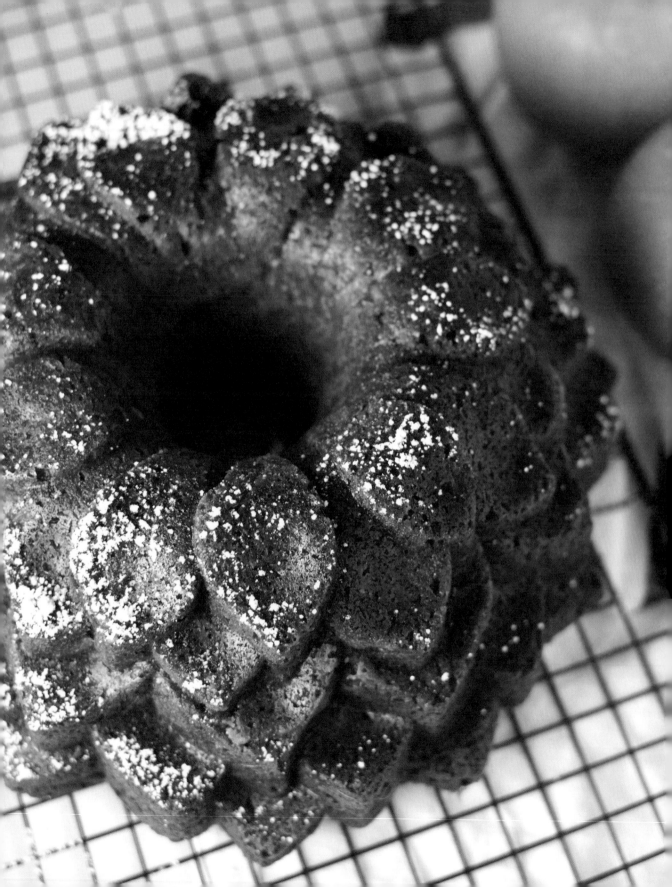

Spiced Honey Apple Cake

RECIPE BY THE DIZZY BAKER • MAKES 8 SERVINGS

When I first got sick, I decided to get back to the basics and cut out all processed food, but I still wanted simple and delicious treats. This sweet and spicy cake fits that bill. It's quick to prepare, full of flavor, and freezes nicely cut into slices for an easy grab-and-go breakfast, snack, or dessert. —JB

---

1 cup unsalted butter, melted (reserve wrappers for greasing the Bundt pan)

3 cups all-purpose flour

½ cup white cane sugar

¼ cup packed light brown sugar

2 teaspoons ground cinnamon

2 teaspoons ground ginger

1 teaspoon baking powder

1 teaspoon baking soda

¾ teaspoon table salt

½ teaspoon ground nutmeg

¼ teaspoon ground cloves

¾ cup honey

3 large eggs

1½ teaspoons vanilla extract

¼ cup natural applesauce (spice- and additive-free)

2–3 Granny Smith or Honeycrisp apples, peeled and grated or minced (about 2 cups)

Powdered sugar for decorating (optional)

Preheat the oven to 350°F. Grease a 10-inch round Bundt cake pan with leftover butter on the wrapper. Take the time to coat every crevice of the inner surface.

In a large bowl, whisk together the flour, white and brown sugars, cinnamon, ginger, baking powder, baking soda, salt, nutmeg, and cloves. Add the melted butter, honey, eggs, and vanilla; mix with an electric mixer on medium speed until well blended. Add the applesauce and grated apples; continue mixing on medium until well combined.

Pour the batter into the prepared pan until it's about ¾ full. Using a rubber spatula, gently push the batter to the edges of the pan and slightly up the walls. Tap the pan on the countertop a few times to help get rid of any air pockets that might interfere with seeing the pretty details of the pan once the cake is unmolded.

Bake the cake until the edges darken and pull away from the sides of the pan and the cake looks slightly browned, 1 hour and 15 minutes. You can be sure it's done by inserting a toothpick into the thickest part of the cake. If it comes out clean, it's ready.

Let the cake cool in the pan for 10 minutes, then invert it onto a wire rack. Tap the pan gently to release the cake. If the cake sticks, carefully use a butter knife to loosen the cake around the edges and center tube, then release again. Cool the unmolded cake for another 10 minutes. When ready to serve, lightly shower the cake with powdered sugar, if desired, and cut into slices.

Ricotta Biscuit Cookies with Vanilla Bean Glaze

RECIPE BY THE DIZZY BAKER • MAKES 4 TO 5 DOZEN COOKIES

If you know me, you know I have a sweet tooth. When I was first diagnosed with vestibular migraine and my neuro-otologist, Dr. Danner, handed me the list of foods I should avoid, I wanted to cry! What would I do to get my cookie fix? I began to scour the internet for chocolate-free cookie recipes and kept coming across a version of these cookies. They were so different from anything I had ever tried before, I couldn't wait to create my own migraine-friendly version. The texture is similar to a biscuit or a scone and they're addictive. I hope you love them as much as I do! —JB

Don't just throw away the used vanilla bean! Once you've removed the vanilla seeds, you can add used vanilla beans to a sugar canister for vanilla-scented sugar. —AW

RICOTTA BISCUIT COOKIES
3¾ cups all-purpose flour
2 teaspoons baking powder
1 teaspoon table salt
1 cup unsalted butter,
   at room temperature
1¾ cups white cane sugar
2 large eggs
15 ounces whole-milk
   ricotta cheese
3 teaspoons vanilla extract

VANILLA BEAN GLAZE
1 vanilla bean
1½ cups powdered sugar
3 tablespoons milk

To make the Ricotta Biscuit Cookies, in a medium bowl, whisk together the flour, baking powder, and salt. In a large bowl, combine the butter and sugar using an electric mixer on medium speed. Add the eggs and mix well. Drain any excess liquid from the ricotta cheese and add it to the butter mixture. Add the vanilla; mix until smooth and creamy. Slowly stir in the flour mixture until blended. Cover the bowl with plastic wrap and refrigerate for at least 1 hour.

Preheat the oven to 350°F. Line 2 baking sheets with parchment paper or silicone baking mats. Drop the dough by heaping tablespoonfuls onto the lined baking sheets, spacing 2 inches apart. Bake until lightly browned on the bottom, 12 to 14 minutes. Transfer cookies to a wire rack and allow them to completely cool before glazing. (They will firm up as they cool.)

To make the Vanilla Bean Glaze, with a sharp paring knife, cut down the length of the vanilla bean, being careful not to cut all the way through. Peel the sides back and use the back of the knife to scrape down the length of the bean, extracting the seed paste. Add the paste to a small bowl. Add the powdered sugar and milk; whisk until smooth.

Spoon the glaze over each cooled cookie and allow to set for about 2 hours before serving.

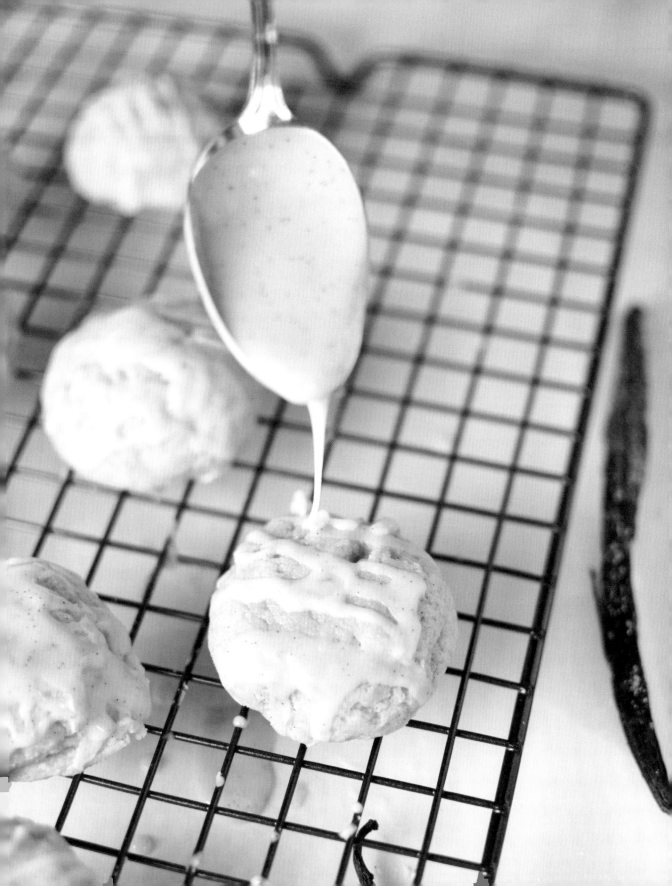

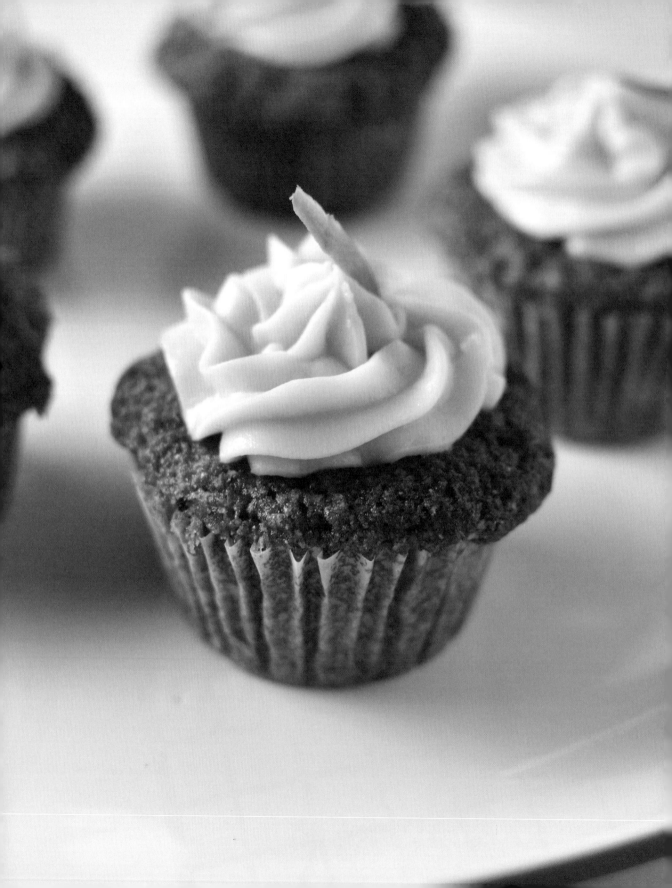

Carrot Cupcakes
with Cream Cheese Frosting

RECIPE BY THE DIZZY BAKER • MAKES 24 CUPCAKES

Spiced goodness isn't just for fall—these cupcakes are also the perfect springtime comfort food. They bring back delightful childhood memories for me with every bite. For example, when I was young, my mom loved to make carrot cake for my family at Easter. I hope this migraine-friendly version of my mom's recipe becomes a springtime tradition for your family as well. Use block cream cheese, not a spreadable variety, for the best frosting texture. —JB

CARROT CUPCAKES
1½ cups all-purpose flour
1½ teaspoons baking soda
1 teaspoon ground cinnamon
¾ teaspoon table salt
¼ teaspoon *each* ground
    nutmeg and ground ginger
¾ cup packed light brown sugar
½ cup granulated sugar
½ cup plus 2 tablespoons
    canola oil or room-
    temperature unsalted butter
⅓ cup unsweetened natural
    applesauce
1½ teaspoons vanilla extract
3 large eggs
1½ cups finely shredded carrots
    (about 3 medium carrots)

CREAM CHEESE FROSTING
½ cup unsalted butter,
    at room temperature
8 ounces cream cheese
    (carrageenan free),
    at room temperature
Pinch of table salt
1½ teaspoons vanilla extract
3–4 cups powdered sugar

To make the Carrot Cupcakes, preheat the oven to 350°F. Line two 12-cup muffin pans with paper liners. In a medium bowl, whisk together the flour, baking soda, cinnamon, salt, nutmeg, and ginger. In a large bowl, combine the brown sugar, granulated sugar, oil or butter, applesauce, and vanilla with an electric mixer on medium-high speed. Add the eggs, one at a time, and continue mixing until smooth. Mix in the carrots, setting aside a few shreds to garnish the cupcakes later. Slowly add the flour mixture to the carrot mixture, mixing until just blended.

Divide batter evenly among cupcake cups, filling ¾ full. Bake until a toothpick inserted into the center comes out mostly clean, about 20 to 22 minutes. Allow the cupcakes to cool completely in the pan before frosting.

To make the Cream Cheese Frosting, beat the butter in a large bowl with an electric mixer on medium-high speed until light and pale. Add the cream cheese, salt, and vanilla. Mix until the mixture is smooth and creamy. Add the powdered sugar 1 cup at a time until the desired consistency is reached. (I typically use 3 cups, which allows for a looser icing. Use closer to 4 cups if you like your icing thick and firm.)

If desired, put the frosting in a piping bag fitted with the decorating tip of your choice. Pipe or spread the frosting onto the cooled cupcakes. Top each with a few carrot shreds and serve.

Simple Watermelon Sorbet

RECIPE BY THE DIZZY BAKER • MAKES 4 SERVINGS

Gluten-, refined sugar–, and dairy-free, this watermelon sorbet is so refreshing and sweet it makes the perfect summer treat. You can swap out watermelon for any safe fruit you like, such as honeydew, peaches, or cherries. Let your imagination run wild and have some fun deciding which flavor you like best. Here's a tip: when freezing the watermelon—or other fruit—before pureeing, be sure the chunks don't touch one another. This helps them not stick together in big chunks, which makes for easier blending. This sorbet is best when eaten immediately. If you refreeze it, chill the container before adding the leftover sorbet to help cut down on ice crystals. And plan to leave it out at room temperature for a few minutes before serving. —JB

3½–4 cups fresh watermelon chunks (about half of a medium-sized watermelon)

2 teaspoons tart cherry or apple juice

1–4 tablespoons warm water, if needed

1 tablespoon honey (optional)

Arrange the watermelon chunks on a wax-paper-lined tray or freezer-safe container, being sure the pieces don't touch each other. A plastic ice cube tray works well too. Freeze overnight.

When ready to serve, place the frozen watermelon pieces in a food processor or high-speed blender, add the cherry or apple juice, and allow to sit 5 minutes. Blend everything together until smooth (a tamper will help if you're using a blender). If the sorbet seems too thick, add warm water 1 tablespoon at a time until you achieve the consistency you're looking for. For a sweeter flavor, blend in a tablespoon of honey. Serve immediately.

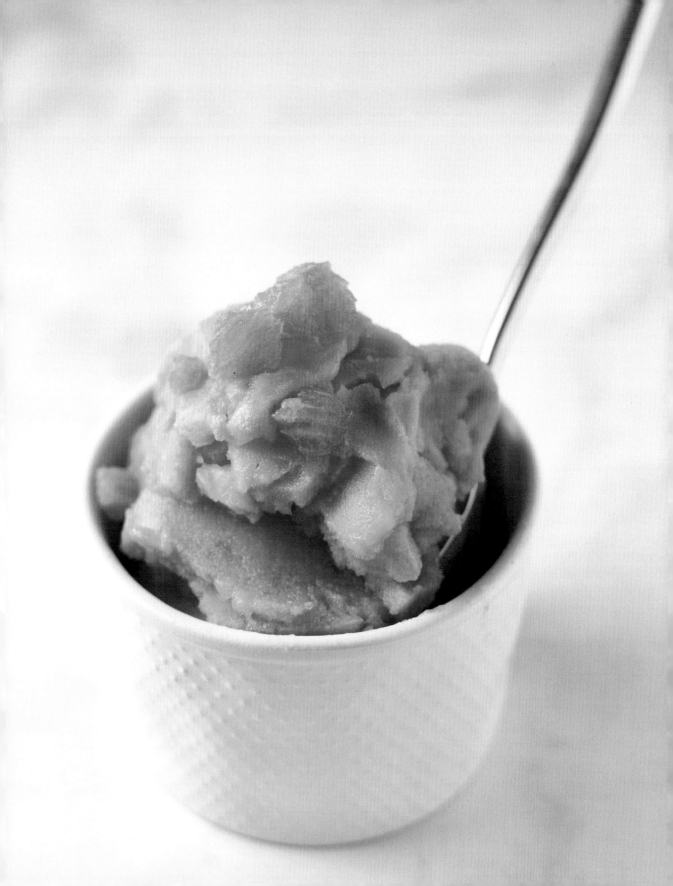

Migraine-Compliant Meal Plans

A little bit of planning is essential to having success with an elimination diet like this one. Stocking pantry staples that are safe and having some quick meals stocked in the freezer will make life so much easier, especially when a migraine attack strikes and there's no energy for cooking. I've put together three detailed meal plans: one for those tough weeks when cooking a big meal sounds miserable, one for those who are looking for migraine-friendly vegetarian options, and one for those who have picky family members. This is just something to get you started, but there are endless combinations in this book.

I also give you ideas for some of my favorite themed meals. As I said previously, I'm a huge fan of having everyone over to my house so I can control the food and the setting. My tailgate meal plan comes in handy during football season, and my friends can never say no to a Tex-Mex meal on our outdoor patio.

When entertaining, I like to invite guests to build their own mocktails. I set out different migraine-friendly juices—such as watermelon, mango, and pomegranate—and a few bottles of plain sparkling water. I also offer fresh herb sprigs for guests to garnish their drinks.

*Denotes recipes that can be made ahead and frozen

TOUGH-WEEK MEAL PLANS

Everyone with a migraine disorder has those days where we struggle to even get out of bed. This is the best meal plan for when you just don't feel like cooking. A lot of these items are simple to put together or can be made ahead and frozen for quick meals. For lunch, you can buy "naked" rotisserie chickens, pick the meat, and freeze it for sandwiches and salads, or use the Anyone-Can-Cook Roast Chicken without the gravy. Many recipes freeze well, so it's a great idea to make them on days you feel good and keep them in the freezer to have just in case. Remember that ginger and turmeric have pain-fighting power, so a warm drink like the Golden Spiced Latte can help ease some symptoms.

BREAKFAST

- Vanilla or Blueberry Chia Pudding (page 57)
- Basic Overnight Oats (page 41)

LUNCH

- Chicken sandwiches or wraps made from Anyone-Can-Cook Roast Chicken* (page 148)
- Farro & Lemongrass Chicken Soup* (page 109)

SNACKS

- Seed Butter Energy Balls* (page 131)
- Apples
- Crackers
- Golden Spiced Latte (page 36) or hot water with fresh ginger

DINNER

- Sheet Pan Salmon, Kale & Potatoes with Dijon-Dill Sauce (page 142) without the sauce
- Slow Cooker or Instant Pot Pulled Pork* (page 153) in a salad, tacos, or quesadillas
- Moroccan Meatballs* (page 138) with couscous, migraine-friendly hummus and pita, or on top of a green salad

VEGETARIAN MEAL PLANS

If you're craving a plant-based menu but still want to be HYH compliant, here's a meal plan for you. For the enchiladas, you can use the Salsa Verde Chicken Enchiladas recipe but substitute some of the vegetable suggestions on the recipe page. The following items can be made ahead, so think of them if you have a busy week coming up: MSG-Free Party Mix, Pepita Protein Bars, Crunchy Buckwheat Granola, Celery Seed and/or Italian Dressing, and Vegetable Broth.

BREAKFAST

- Crunchy Buckwheat Granola (page 45)
- Nutty Pancakes (page 65)
- Faux-Yo Açaí Bowl (page 42)
- SB&J Smoothie (page 62)

LUNCH

- Curried Carrot & Sweet Potato Soup (page 102) made with Vegetable Broth* (page 80)
- Summer Pasta Salad with Zesty Herb Dressing (page 90)
- Chilled Soba Noodle Salad (page 93)
- Baked Bean Taquitos (page 58)

SNACKS

- Pepita Protein Bars* (page 116)
- MSG-Free Party Mix (page 127)

DINNER

- Vegetarian Enchiladas* (variation of Salsa Verde Chicken Enchiladas, page 137)
- Pumpkin Sage Pasta (page 150)
- Mexican-Style Stuffed Sweet Potatoes (page 145)
- Winter Rice Pilaf (page 172) and a giant salad tossed with Celery Seed Dressing (page 72)
- Spinach Artichoke Flatbreads (page 124) and a side salad tossed with Italian Dressing (page 70)

FAMILY-FRIENDLY MEAL PLANS

These are the recipes I consider to be total crowd pleasers. For families on the go, store the Sausage Balls and Pepita Protein Bars in the freezer for a quick meal you can eat as you run out the door. As a Dr. Seuss fan, I hope the kids will love Green Eggs No Ham. I know my mom could convince me to eat anything if it came with tortilla chips. For the sandwiches, I like to spread a little bit of Boursin Garlic & Fine Herbs cheese on some good bread, then add chicken or veggies like roasted red peppers, cucumber, lettuce, and radishes.

BREAKFAST

- Leek & Goat Cheese Breakfast Casserole (page 54)
- Sausage Balls* (page 53)
- Pepita Protein Bars* (page 116)
- Green Eggs No Ham (Shakshuka Verde) (page 46)

LUNCH

- Chicken or vegetable sandwiches (see note above)
- Big salad tossed with Southwestern Ranch Dressing (page 70)

DINNER

- Salsa Verde Chicken Enchiladas* (page 137), (or the same filling made with the Enchilada Sauce on page 79) and Mexican-Style Black Beans* (page 187), and a side salad with Southwestern Ranch Dressing (page 70)
- Mini Barbecue Meatloaves* (page 146) with Whipped Parsnips (page 183) or simple mashed potatoes
- Mediterranean-Style Baked Halibut (page 154) with roasted potatoes and broccoli
- Grilled Chipotle Steak Fajita Bowls (page 157)

OTHER MEAL IDEAS:

WHEN YOU NEED A VACATION
- Pomegranate Nojito (page 32)
- Maui Kale Salad (page 86)
- Seared Sea Scallops with Mango Salsa (page 166)

DATE NIGHT
- Garlic Spinach & Tomatoes (page 180)
- Mac & Fresh Cheese (page 175)
- Anyone-Can-Cook Roast Chicken* with Rosemary Gravy (page 148)

HOLIDAY ITEMS
- Leek & Goat Cheese Breakfast Casserole (page 54)
- Bruschetta Board (page 120)
- Burrata, Corn & Arugula Salad with Za'atar Croutons (page 101)
- Boursin Scalloped Potatoes (page 188)
- Lamb Chops with Cilantro Chimichurri (page 165)

TAILGATE
- Smoky Carrot Hummus (page 119)
- MSG-Free Party Mix (page 127)
- Crispy Taco-Spiced Chicken Wings (page 132)
- Slow-Cooker or Instant Pot Pulled Pork* (page 153) with Barbecue Sauce (page 75)

DINNER WITH FRIENDS
- Queso Dip (page 115)
- Mexican-Style Black Beans* (page 187)
- Salsa Verde Chicken Enchiladas* (page 137) or improvised enchiladas made with Slow Cooker or Instant Pot Pulled Pork* (page 153)
- Black & Blue Sunflower Seed Crumble (page 197)

GRILLING NIGHT
- Chipotle steak from Grilled Chipotle Steak Fajita Bowls (page 157)
- Smoky Sweet Potatoes (page 171)
- Charred Corn & Farro Summer Salad (page 89)

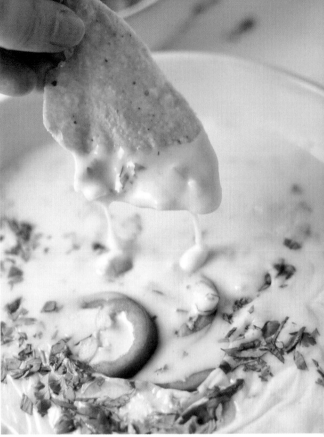

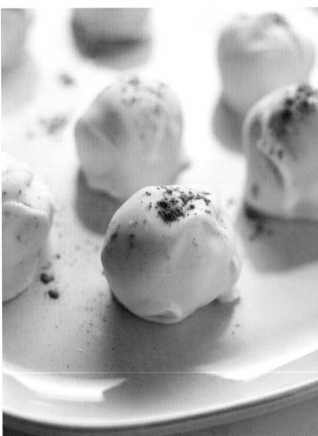

Vestibular Migraine: More Than a Headache

There are quite a few books available for migraine, but they rarely mention vestibular migraine. The ones that do refer to it don't go into much detail. This could be because it's only been recognized as a diagnosis in the past ten years, and many doctors are still not aware that it exists. Often, they are more familiar with other vestibular disorders like Meniere's disease or BPPV, which have similar symptoms. Many doctors who are not familiar with vestibular disorders often overlook small factors that separate one diagnosis from another. Despite its prevalence, accounting for roughly 10 percent of migraine patients (likely higher in reality due to misdiagnosis), a diagnosis of VM is based on the exclusion of other causes of dizziness. This disorder has impacted my life so much, and I feel it's important to include a primer in this book about what I've learned regarding symptoms and treatments, in order to help others on their journey.

VESTIBULAR MIGRAINE SYMPTOMS

Many people, like myself prior to my diagnosis, think of migraine as horrible head pain, sensitivity to light, and nausea, among other symptoms. What people don't realize is that it's possible to have vestibular migraine without any head pain. Less than half of patients actually experience a link between vertigo and headache. With vestibular migraine, while head pain is still possible, the most common symptoms involve dissociation, visual disturbances, lightheadedness, ataxia (impaired coordination), giddiness, a floaty feeling, or rotational spinning (vertigo). Some refer to vestibular migraine as "MAV" or "Migraine Associated Vertigo," but I believe this is a confusing term because some patients with vestibular migraine never actually experience a vertigo attack. In most physicians' minds, vertigo strictly references a rotational spinning sensation that usually leads to vomiting.

Other symptoms involve light sensitivity, tinnitus (ear ringing), head pressure, disequilibrium, and visual distortions. Some days I felt like I was on a boat that was rocking side to side or up and down. Restaurants were so difficult because all my senses were heightened. A flickering candle, loud music, or a boisterous conversation would make my head feel super fuzzy, as if I couldn't focus on any one thing. The brain fog was so terrible, I had a tough time recalling my best friends' names or basic objects in a conversation. Previously I had a quick wit, but with VM it was challenging to form a basic sentence.

It's important to be able to describe your symptoms accurately so your doctor can give you the best diagnosis. I worked with Dr. Edward Cho from House Clinic in Los Angeles to define these terms in more detail so that patients can accurately describe their symptoms to their physicians. Being descriptive and precise in what you say will not only help your doctor formulate the correct diagnosis but can also help with your treatment plan. Here are some of the symptoms defined:

Vertigo–a feeling of motion when there is no motion. Most commonly associated with spinning, where you feel you are spinning, or your surroundings are spinning. Dr. Cho says physicians understand vertigo as primarily spinning to keep it distinguishable from other symptoms. Physicians will ask you to describe your type of vertigo and note if the episodes are continuous or if they are short bursts.

They will also want to know if the vertigo episode is positional (based on how you move) or if it happens spontaneously. These questions can help your physician narrow the type of vertigo. There are two types of vertigo: peripheral and central.

Peripheral Vertigo–associated with short bursts of rotational spinning. Nystagmus—involuntary, rapid eye movements—can be horizontal or rotational, and the presence of vertigo when you wake up in the morning suggests peripheral vertigo. It is common with other vestibular disorders like Meniere's, BPPV, and Labyrinthitis or Vestibular Neuronitis. These disorders cause vertigo "outside the brain," usually originating from the inner ear.

Central Vertigo—originates from the brain and can last much longer than peripheral vertigo, from hours to days. It's the type of vertigo typically associated with migraine.

Lightheadedness—a sensation just short of fainting (a physician may refer to this as near syncope or presyncope). Sometimes you can feel this from standing up quickly or along with heavy breathing. You may feel as if you're about to pass out or can't get enough air.

Disequilibrium—a sensation associated with being unstable on your feet. This is the feeling of walking on clouds or like the ground is moving up and down beneath you, perhaps like you're on a boat. This may also fit a rocking, tilting, and/or swaying description.

Anxiety—associated with worry or fear of performing certain tasks. You may feel panicked or have quickness of breath.

Giddiness—probably the best description of what we think of when we use the word "dizziness." It's a reeling sensation, and you may feel like you're about to fall.

Depersonalization—a disconnection from your body; feeling separated either from yourself or your surroundings, almost like you're in a dream or trapped in a bubble. You might feel weightless, or like your head might "pop" off and float away.

Derealization—disconnection from the environment around you. You may feel like you're looking at the world from behind a window or veil. Or there is an alteration of the world around you that seems unreal. The space and size of things around you may be altered. This is also called "Alice in Wonderland syndrome." Dr. Cho mentions that derealization is one of the symptoms he sees often, but patients either don't fully describe these symptoms to their doctors or don't know how. Perhaps they believe they are "losing their minds" and don't want others to think they're going crazy. These symptoms are very common with migraine, vestibular disorders, and epilepsy.

Visual Dependence and Visual Motion—when your vision is not matching up with what is actually going on with the world around you, it can create dizziness. For instance, you may be parked in the car, but feel like you or the cars around you are moving when they're not. With visual dependence, you may be putting more weight on your sight rather than leaning on other forms of balance—like the inner ear, feet, and spatial recognition. If scrolling on your smartphone or computer drives you nuts, or you cannot tolerate driving or being in grocery stores, you probably have this symptom. This can also be associated with PPPD.

Tinnitus—a ringing or buzzing in the ears. It can also manifest as hissing, chirping, or several other sounds—sporadic or continuous.

Ataxia—feeling "drunk" or having difficulty walking (gait abnormality). You might have slurred speech, stumble, or have a lack of coordination. It's similar to disequilibrium.

Photophobia—light sensitivity. Sunlight, fluorescent light, and incandescent light can all trigger this issue. It may cause discomfort, increased symptoms, or the need to squint/close your eyes. You may want to wear sunglasses indoors.

Smell Sensitivity—certain scents, especially strong candles or lotions, can trigger an immediate reaction.

Motion Sickness or Sensitivity (Kinesiophobia)—the feeling of nausea or the increase in other symptoms from riding in cars, on a plane, or even scrolling through your smartphone.

Phonophobia—sensitivity to sound, where music, loud conversations, or other noises seem very harsh. Hyperacusis is an extreme form of phonophobia but is less common.

The process of exclusion for diagnosing vestibular migraine involves a hearing test to rule out hearing loss (common with Meniere's), a family history (migraine is widely genetic), an MRI, caloric testing, and VNG/ENG tests that look for slow saccades (an abnormal speed of eye movement) and nystagmus (repetitive, uncontrollable eye movements). VM patients often find that their MRIs return with normal results but may show white spots that are different from the white matter lesions that show up for a multiple sclerosis patient. It is also possible for Meniere's patients to have crossover with vestibular migraine, making both vestibular disorders even more difficult to diagnose.

VESTIBULAR THERAPY & DIET

Physicians sometimes recommend that patients who are incredibly sensitive to motion or certain stimuli try vestibular rehabilitation therapy, also known as VRT. This entails performing exercises that allow the brain to compensate for certain movements. The idea is that the brain will learn to accept these movements without triggering dizziness. In my case, I truly believe VRT helped once I wasn't suffering from 24/7 symptoms. The key was to find a therapist who was knowledgeable about vestibular migraine. Previously I had gone to therapists who never mentioned a "baseline" and just pushed me through a grueling therapy session. A "baseline" is the level of dizziness you are at before you start any exercise. When being pushed to my limit, I always felt worse after and never really saw improvement. Once my symptoms were slightly more well controlled on medication, supplements, and the HYH diet, I saw a new vestibular therapist who explained to me that it's important to always return to that "baseline" of when you started. Your symptoms should only be briefly elevated, for no more than an hour.

An interesting exercise that we tried was to prepare me for a trip to Las Vegas after being diagnosed. Vegas was one of the first places I visited after being diagnosed and it was probably the worst place for someone with a vestibular disorder. The flashing lights, loud noises, odd smells, and crazy carpets were all too much, and I spent the majority of the trip in the hotel room. When I discussed my anxiety about returning to the city with my therapist, she had me watch YouTube videos of people walking through Vegas casinos. There were levels I could work up to depending on how I felt. Easy would be considered a professional video that's shot with a camera stabilizer. Difficult would be some drunk guy walking around filming with his iPhone while holding a beer and shouting at his kids. After watching these videos over several months, my second trip to Vegas was much more successful than my first.

As far as diet, many specialists, like Dr. Michael Teixido who was interviewed for the 2019 Migraine World Summit's inaugural talk specifically about vestibular migraine, agree that a low-tyramine, additive-free migraine diet can have a positive effect on decreasing attacks and improving vestibular migraine. The most effective clinics are implementing a multimodal approach of treating any chronic illness to bring an increased chance of success to patients. These physicians recognize that personal treatment can vary, but combining a diet full of whole foods, various types of therapy, alternative remedies, exercise, and medication when needed is widely useful for migraine patients. Be sure to consult your trusted healthcare team and family to find the path that's right for you.

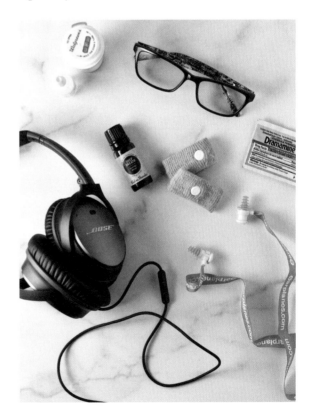

Alternative Treatments for Migraine:
The Magic Pill Does Not Exist

There's not one single migraine diet out there that will be the answer to all your problems. For me, and for most people, it's a combination of treatments that helps break the migraine cycle. My favorite online support group, Migraine Strong, calls this "The Treatment Pie." The pie is made up of medication, supplements, movement, diet, sleep, therapy, hydration, mindfulness, and a free slice of whatever you think might work well for you. This could be anything from acupuncture to massage. I've heard that acupuncture was the answer for so many people, but I didn't notice that it helped me, and that's okay. I found out that my body responds much better to acupressure and reflexology.

Just because a part of the pie didn't make a difference for one person does not mean it won't be the missing piece that makes a huge difference for you. It's also important to note that some people need medication in addition to natural treatments. Sometimes natural treatments are not enough on their own, but they can assist with some of the heavy lifting that the medication does. Needing medication does not make you a failure. All these pie slices work together to decrease our overall threshold of that point where a migraine attack begins. I see people who comment that a diet or certain supplements never helped them, but I think what some fail to realize is that the changes are incremental. Adding

THE TREATMENT PIE

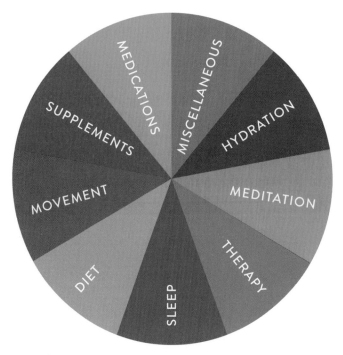

The Treatment Pie
courtesy of Migraine Strong

one supplement is not likely to transform your life overnight. It takes time, discipline, and a little bit of hope that these things are all working together to bring that threshold down.

SUPPLEMENTS

Supplements are the most studied of all the natural treatments that are available for migraine. Your doctor has most likely mentioned that you should try magnesium, riboflavin (B2), and CoQ10. All three supplements have been proven to be effective preventatives. The Johns Hopkins Headache Center patient handout of vitamins and dietary supplements for migraine recommends their patients start with 400 milligrams of B2, 600 to 800 milligrams of magnesium, and 100–300 milligrams of CoQ10. The B2 and CoQ10 are straightforward, but what happens when you go to buy a magnesium supplement and you have a thousand different kinds to try? Are some better than others? Actually, yes.

Migraine disorders can be linked with magnesium

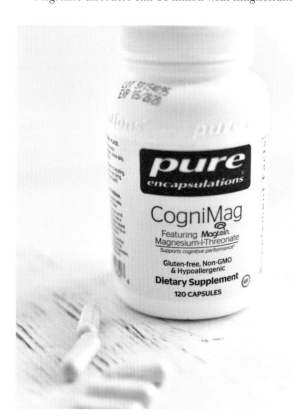

deficiency, making supplementation necessary for most of us. However, if you're finding that you have more digestive "issues" when upping your magnesium intake, you're not alone. I wasn't aware until I started doing a little more research after my combination migraine supplement was giving me stomach cramps and loose stools. I realized that the magnesium in this supplement was more commonly prescribed as a laxative… something I did not need.

When people search for a new magnesium supplement without knowing what to look for, they usually focus on price. That means many aren't getting the full potential out of the supplements they're taking. This could be because our body doesn't agree with that form of magnesium. Or it could be that the supplement contains additional fillers or potential migraine triggers, making it poor quality and more difficult to absorb. *Holy Water, Sacred Oil: The Fountain of Youth* by C. Norman Shealy mentions that magnesium is most effective when contained in the intestine for a minimum of 12 hours. If magnesium is going through the system faster (i.e., in the form of diarrhea), you are not getting the full benefits of the supplement you're taking.

One key word to know is "bioavailability," which means how well the supplement is absorbed by the body. If the supplement you're taking is not very bioavailable, it's not being metabolized and you're most likely not reaping the benefits from it. As we age and our metabolism slows, it can be even more important to focus on bioavailability, as vitamins can become more difficult to absorb. Therefore, choosing high-quality supplements is paramount. Fillers, binders, and artificial ingredients or flavorings can all limit absorption. Magnesium itself isn't a highly absorbable supplement to begin with, but if you have a deficiency, your body will be able to take in more than it would otherwise.

You also want to make sure you don't take calcium or a multivitamin at the same time as the magnesium supplements. Certain supplements, like calcium, compete with absorption of magnesium. If taken together, you could be hindering magnesium from being fully absorbed by your body.

A MIGRAINE SUFFERER'S GUIDE TO SUPPLEMENTS

Before you take any supplements or any other health remedy, be sure to check with your doctor to be sure this treatment is right for your individual circumstances. A doctor will also recommend individualized dosages customized for your personal treatment plan. The following supplements are generally considered to be part of a migraine sufferer's arsenal of potential tools to prevent migraine symptoms.

MAGNESIUM GLYCINATE This type of magnesium is one of the most effective at boosting low levels of magnesium quickly, without causing digestive problems or diarrhea. It is ideal for those who cannot tolerate the laxative effects of citrate or oxide and need a more well-absorbed form. Because migraine patients are recommended to take around 600 to 800 milligrams of magnesium daily, glycinate can be added for higher supplementation. Glycine, an amino acid to which the magnesium is bonded, supports cognitive function and calms neural functions while elevating serotonin levels. Therefore, patients find this form helps with reducing inflammation, improving sleep quality, and lowering anxiety. For those with vestibular migraine, which is often connected to slow cognitive function and anxiety, this could be a great fit.

MAGNESIUM L-THREONATE A newer type of magnesium, this is one of the only forms of magnesium that has been shown to penetrate the blood brain barrier, directly raising magnesium levels in the brain. In studies, it played a positive role with improving Alzheimer's and other cognitive issues. Developed by MIT graduates, Magtein (a branded form of Magnesium L-Threonate) promotes improvement of learning abilities, memory, and cognitive function. It even helped me get rid of my morning brain fog, a common symptom with vestibular migraine. I've had several people tell me that taking this gives them the same alertness and mental clarity that they would get from a cup of coffee. This type also doesn't contain laxative properties that you would find with citrate or oxide. The downside? It's expensive and fairly new, so there's not as much known about it. Threonate is a good one to supplement in addition to another form of magnesium so you're saving money and reaping benefits from both.

MAGNESIUM CHLORIDE & MAGNESIUM SULFATE You might be more familiar with Epsom salts, also known as magnesium sulfate. Through research and discussion with other migraine patients, it seems as if magnesium chloride is like Epsom salt on steroids. It appears to have better absorption and cellular penetration, as well as lower tissue toxicity. This form of magnesium is wonderful for topical applications, especially if you'd like to supplement your oral intake. This would include adding it to a bath, foot soak, or lotion. Concentration of the solution, length of time it is in contact with the skin, and area where it is applied all affect magnesium chloride's efficacy. Some find that if they do a soak for 20 to 30 minutes or apply to their feet before bed, it helps to calm the body and promote a deeper sleep, but there's not a lot of solid scientific research to back these claims.

MAGNESIUM MALATE Some patients with migraine also suffer from fibromyalgia and chronic fatigue syndrome, making magnesium malate a good choice. It's a combination of malic acid and magnesium, which is said to have a higher bioavailability. Another positive is that it supports energy production and promotes the ability to remove toxic metals that build up in the body. Malate also creates less GI stress than citrate and oxide. The only downside is that some find this form too energizing, so it's a good idea to take it in the morning. It also could potentially be too stimulating for those with vestibular migraine.

MAGNESIUM CITRATE One of the most popular and well-studied forms of magnesium, this type bonds to citric acid, making it highly absorbable. If you Google "magnesium citrate," you'll notice it's promoted to relieve constipation, which is helpful (sometimes!). However, if you're taking this at the recommended amounts each day (600 to 800 milligrams), you could be spending long mornings on the toilet. This means you're probably not getting many benefits from it in the end. Citrate is one of those "proceed with caution" items. If you can tolerate it well in high amounts, great! If you can't, investigate malate, glycinate, or threonate. Citrate mixes well with liquids and could be an option for those who cannot tolerate pills.

MAGNESIUM OXIDE A widely prescribed form of magnesium, this type is cheap and easily found, but it may not be the best option for migraine. Initial studies on migraine and magnesium used magnesium oxide, but that's most likely because it is so widely available and inexpensive. While magnesium citrate can relieve constipation, oxide is commonly used to relieve heartburn and indigestion (as well as constipation). It is not as bioavailable as magnesium citrate or some of the other forms. If you've been taking this form and not seeing results, there are better options that could be more highly effective.

MAGNESIUM TAURATE

Taurate, the amino acid taurine combined with magnesium, is another well-studied form of magnesium. It has been shown to reduce heart attacks and promote stable blood sugar levels. In studies, taurate was highly effective in migraine prevention while having limited side effects. If you also have cardiovascular issues, this could be a good choice for you.

RIBOFLAVIN (B2)

In my first appointment, Dr. Beh told me this is one of the best vitamins for migraine. It has been scientifically proven that it works well for migraine prevention, even for children. Like magnesium, people with chronic migraine may be B2 deficient. What's interesting to me is B2 deficiency has side effects of digestive problems. I had struggled with IBS symptoms before my vestibular migraine disease began, which I attributed to stress, but my issues have cleared after starting the supplements and diet. Studies using 400 milligrams of B2 have shown that it can cut the number of headache days in half, reducing the amount of triptans used. Some studies showed reduction in the length and severity of migraine. Riboflavin is relatively inexpensive and has minimal risk of side effects, although it does interact with certain medications like some tricyclic anti-depressants. Therefore, it's best to have your physician's approval first on any new supplements.

CoQ10

In medical trials, 100 milligrams of CoQ10 proved to be effective at decreasing overall attack days, as well as minimizing pain and nausea. Patients who benefited from CoQ10 also had shorter attacks than previously noted. Overall, it is a well-tolerated supplement that could be beneficial for those who struggle with brain fog, memory problems, and mental clarity. The only downside is that a good CoQ10 without a lot of fillers can be quite expensive. A less expensive option is feverfew, a plant in the daisy family. While I personally haven't had luck with feverfew, it has been effective for some of my friends with migraine. It appears to be better when taken to abort a migraine attack rather than as a daily preventative.

GINGER

The ultimate pain-fighting natural treatment, ginger is an effective way to thwart an attack. Studies have shown that just ⅛ teaspoon of ground ginger can be as effective at aborting head pain as Sumatriptan (Imitrex). Within just 2 hours of taking ginger, head pain was significantly decreased for study participants. Plus, there's no risk of rebound associated with ginger like there is for triptans. For those with vestibular migraine, not only can ginger help to ease an attack, but it can also soothe the stomach from the nausea that's commonly associated. One side effect that I tend to get from ginger is heartburn, so I find it's best to mix the powder in with smoothies or other food items. You can also take it as a supplement with food.

FILLERS, GELATIN & BINDING AGENTS

One last thing to keep in mind when searching for magnesium supplements for migraine is fillers, gelatin, and binding agents. Supplements, like food, should contain very few ingredients. If you see a long list, it could be that the supplement contains very little elemental value, with more fillers to "bulk" it up. Some of these include cellulose, magnesium stearate, and stearic acid. In the end, you won't save much money if you're not absorbing the supplement well.

I recommend people search for vegan capsules, which tend to have fewer ingredients and also use vegetable cellulose over gelatin. For some people who are highly sensitive to glutamate, they find that even the smallest gelatin capsule can be triggering. If you notice your symptoms increasing after taking supplements, it's worth looking at the label to see if it's a filler that could be causing the symptoms and not the supplement itself.

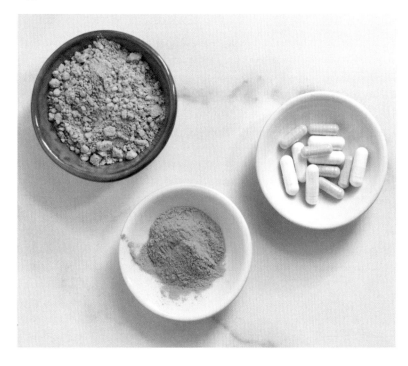

EXERCISE & MIGRAINE

Physical activity is important for most patients with migraine because of the release of endorphins, which help with pain. A study from 2011 by Varkey, Cider, Carlsson, and Lindy showed exercising at least 3 times a week for 40 minutes per session was as effective as relaxation techniques and preventative use of Topamax.

If you can't even imagine leaving your bed right now, trust me, I've been there. Starting slow is okay, and this is where goal setting can come into play. Your first goal may be to walk to the mailbox. Once you feel confident in that, try walking down the street, then maybe around the block. When you get to a place where you'd like to advance your exercise routine, I highly recommend beginner ballet classes. On my first day of class, I walked into the studio so nervous, but I explained my illness to the instructor, and we worked on modifying the class to fit my needs. Over time, I built up my balance and got more confident to do strenuous workouts. I know that intense exercises like HIIT classes will trigger symptoms for me, but I always return to my baseline within the hour. To me, this is a sign that I can get through a difficult class while still improving my vestibular system through exercise.

Many doctors suggested yoga to me, but I found that sun salutations were my worst enemy in the beginning. Moving my head up and down so quickly left me dizzy and unbalanced. I almost threw in the towel (no pun intended), when I finally tried restorative yoga. With restorative yoga, you still use some balance, but the movements are slow and more like a deep stretch. It also includes mindfulness and breathing techniques, which can transfer into your everyday life. There are many YouTube videos out there with examples and poses so you can see if it's the right fit for you before you sign up for a class. Always let the instructor know about your illness. Not only will it increase awareness, but it can also give a boost of confidence knowing that someone else is watching out for you.

THERAPY, MINDFULNESS & MEDITATION

Any kind of migraine can come with increased anxiety. Growing up, I was always a little stressed or anxious. I have an overachiever personality. But my anxiety became overwhelming when this chronic illness hit. Suddenly I was terrified to drive or even leave the house. You want to do everything possible not to have those symptoms spike. However, this mentality can lead to depression. Many of us are often hit out of nowhere and must leave our jobs to focus on our health, or your employer might find a way to let you go. It is soul crushing because you're terrified for yourself and for your livelihood. Since there's no magic pill, you're left to try all these treatments and wonder when you'll improve. This is why it's often necessary to seek counseling.

Counseling doesn't always have to be expensive. In fact, my insurance plan covered a certain number of sessions for me and even offered free counselors over the phone. There are also counseling apps where you can speak to someone from the comfort of your home. If you find yourself in a position where you're sad all the time, it's okay to reach out for help. Your counselor can teach you techniques to help you stay calm in the midst of an attack. They can also help you with the goal setting that I mentioned earlier.

Cognitive Behavioral Therapy (CBT) is recommended for many patients with chronic illness, because it can help you be aware of negative thoughts and teach you how to shift your focus. This allows us to realize the connection between thoughts, emotions, and behaviors. It takes internal events (like dizziness or pain) and external events (your HR department questioning the time you take off for migraine attacks) and helps you recognize them, so your thoughts can produce a calm emotion rather than an anxious one. So instead of having dizziness or pain and immediately thinking, "Oh my gosh, not another attack!" which leads to panic and frustration, you would instead learn to react with, "This is just a sensation and I am okay."

I often take advantage of meditation apps and restorative yoga classes. Focusing on my breathing for just a few minutes makes me realize how often

I hold my breath, not even realizing it. When I feel my dizziness kick in, a few deep breaths in 5-second intervals (5 in, hold for 5, 5 out) can really help calm the mind and bring that anxiety down a few notches. Now when I fly, I listen to a guided meditation or a hemi-sync playlist during takeoff and landing. (Hemi-sync uses binaural beats, a soundwave therapy that guides the brain into a state of relaxation or mindfulness.)

SLEEP & MIGRAINE

This is one area that can, for the most part, be easily controlled, yet we often forget how important sleep is. When I was first diagnosed with vestibular migraine, I was exhausted all the time. I felt as if my eyes were working overtime to try to keep my body steady. Naps became a daily occurrence for me. What I didn't realize was how important a strict sleep schedule is to migraine prevention.

A 2016 study showed that restorative sleep that is at least 7 to 8 hours long can reduce migraine attacks. The overwhelming agreement is that napping takes away from quality sleep at night. It's also important that we maintain a strict sleep cycle: going to bed and waking up within 30 minutes of our usual time, even on weekends. I do find that if I stick to my sleep schedule, my symptoms don't kick up as often as they do when I either don't get enough sleep, go to bed way too late, or take a nap.

CAFFEINE & MIGRAINE

This diet requires you to give up caffeine, which I believe is one of the hardest parts. If you have vestibular migraine, this is especially important as it seems our brains are extremely sensitive to it. Over the years, I slowly became a coffee lover. It didn't help that we had a Starbucks in our office, and it was my one opportunity to get away from my desk. Not to mention my husband considers himself a coffee connoisseur (I would probably replace the word "connoisseur" with "addict"), but that's another story. Coffee has turned into a way of life for most humans, with all the cute shops popping up in every neighborhood. It's a fun, quick way to meet up with

friends, or a good opportunity for networking. It's a nice way to spend a Saturday morning. Now when people ask me to meet for coffee, I literally don't know what to do with myself. Do I explain that it gives me horrible vestibular migraine symptoms? Do I just go and have water? Do I just sit there and try to figure out something to do with my hands?!

I have some alternatives that aren't just tea. In fact, tea can be a huge trigger for me as well. In the beginning of my migraine diet journey, I would even have an issue with naturally caffeine-free teas that are acceptable, like chamomile tea. But let's start with why coffee should be one of the first migraine triggers that you give up.

You may think caffeine is a good migraine fix. It's an essential component of Excedrin Migraine, after all. I've even seen it recommended on Pinterest posts for "curing a migraine." (P.S. Don't ever take migraine "cure" advice from Pinterest or you'll end up with a banana peel on the head.) This is because caffeine has a stimulant effect that opens blood vessels in the brain, allowing for some relief of a headache. Although it can be an effective abortive when used sparingly, it's not a permanent solution. Drinking large amounts of caffeinated coffee every day can even lead to rebound headaches.

There's still conflicting information on this subject, which is understandable considering the incredible dependency on caffeine that we all tend to have. In my opinion, people make excuses to have it around because they are so addicted to it, and it's unimaginable to give up. In my case, I was so desperate to feel normal again that I gave up all my favorite things: aged cheese, red wine, and even my morning latte.

At first, I switched to regular decaf, thinking I was doing something good for myself, but my vestibular symptoms like giddiness would increase after each cup. I found out that there's still a decent amount of caffeine in most decaf coffees, and many of them are processed with chemicals, also leaving a funky aftertaste. The chemical solvents used can leave a residue on the beans, and decaf coffees are only regulated to be 97 percent caffeine free by the USDA.

A typical cup of coffee contains between 70 and 140 milligrams of caffeine, whereas regular decaf can only contain 0 to 7 milligrams. It may not sound like a large amount, but if you already have a sensitive brain, it can trigger symptoms almost immediately.

One thing to note is not to quit cold turkey if your body is used to having it every day. Try mixing your regular coffee with Swiss Water decaf and gradually decreasing the amount over the course of a few weeks. Initially you may have an increase in symptoms, but it should level our with time.

Not All Decafs Are Equal

Coffee is decaffeinated using four different methods, all performed before roasting while the bean is still green. Water, by itself, cannot decaffeinate the bean without washing away other soluble substances like sugar and protein. A decaffeinating agent must be added to aid in the process. There are four different agents used: activated charcoal and CO_2 being natural, and methylene chloride and ethyl acetate being chemical solvents.

Ethyl acetate is actually considered a more "natural" solvent because it can be found organically in ripening fruits. This raised a red flag for me, because ripening fruits can be a powerful migraine trigger for some. Because this solvent can be found in nature, producers can mark the bags as "naturally decaffeinated," even though the chemical used is actually synthetic. All of this is to say that even with coffee, you should check the labels! Just because one says "naturally decaffeinated" or "water processed" does not mean that it is done with the same standards as Swiss Water Process or does not contain chemical solvents.

Swiss Water Process (SWP) coffee was invented in the 1930s and brought to market in the 1980s. The SWP method relies on osmosis to decaffeinate the beans. Beans are first soaked in very hot water to remove the caffeine, then the water is passed through an activated charcoal filter. Larger caffeine molecules are caught in the filter and the flavors we discussed before are allowed to pass through. The caffeine-free beans are then discarded, and the flavored water that passed through is used to soak the next batch of beans being decaffeinated, adding the rich flavor. Cool, right? Swiss Water Process coffee is highly regulated and consistently audited to make sure it is 99.9 percent caffeine free. You'll find it used most often with organic coffees. To check and see if you have a good brand near you, you can go to swisswater.com and use the store locator. I was able to find coffee shops near my home that sell certified Swiss Water Process coffee, so I don't always have to brew a cup myself.

CO_2 process, the other chemical-solvent-free process, also starts by soaking the beans, but then places them in a stainless-steel container to extract the caffeine using liquid CO_2. Because it is lower cost than Swiss Water Process, you'll find this method most often used in large-batch, commercial-grade coffees. Lavazza is a brand that typically uses CO_2 decaffeination.

Other Coffee Alternatives

There are a lot of natural "coffee" blends out there that have nothing to do with beans and more to do with roots or mushrooms. Chicory root has a dark and deep flavor that many describe as nutty. When coffee was scarce in 18th century France, chicory was used as a replacement, and continued to be added to coffee in the 19th century as it was believed to have health benefits. You'll still find chicory-blended coffee in New Orleans, notably at the famous Cafe du Monde. Chicory is often added with other natural additions like dandelion or carob for added flavor. Carob is a gray area on migraine diets, so it's one of those "proceed with caution" items. If you're in a chronic state, it's best to avoid carob. You must be careful with chicory coffee and other coffee substitutes like Teeccino because they may contain triggering ingredients.

You might find that you don't even need a coffee substitute once you give it up for a while. The Golden Spiced Latte might be your new favorite thing. No? That will never happen in this lifetime? Okay, find some Swiss Water Decaf coffee, stat.

Migraine-Savvy Travel Tips

Since my vestibular migraine disorder began after a few weeks of heavy traveling, I was terrified to fly for a long time. It didn't help that one of the first physicians I saw speculated that I had a perilymph fistula and urged me to never fly again. Traveling and discovering new places was a huge part of who I was, and I felt like VM was stealing that from me. It took a conscious decision not to let this rule my life and overcome my fear of flying.

Yet I understand the stress associated with being away from the comfort of home, where you can control the settings. It is a hassle to pack an extra bag of essential oils, rescue meds, and migraine-safe snacks. But with a little planning, you get used to it and it eventually becomes second nature. The extra work is worth the payout of living life to its fullest, even with an illness like migraine.

I'm not going to lie: my first couple of trips were rough. But over time, it got much easier. Now I take international flights without any fear! Here are some things I have learned about traveling with a migraine disorder.

Pressure changes can wreak havoc on sensitive ears. I never fly without EarPlanes. They're small earplugs that help regulate the pressure, making flights a little more enjoyable. You insert them before the cabin door closes and remove them after it's been opened. If it's a long flight, you can remove them at cruising altitude and reinsert them before the descent. Sometimes the adult size can hurt my ears on a long flight, so I use the child's size. Flonase and Afrin can also help keep your eustachian tubes clear.

Sea-Bands are wristbands that trigger an acupressure point, easing nausea and motion sickness. They help to a certain extent, although there's nothing that can overcome a bumpy descent or a lot of turbulence. Before takeoff, double check that there's a "barf bag" in the seatback pocket.

Work with your physician to come up with a rescue plan that works for you. Certain benzodiazepines are frequently recommended as rescue meds when traveling with a vestibular disorder.

As vestibular suppressants, they take the edge off the excitability of travel and also help with anxiety. In the past, it was thought that these medications can affect vestibular compensation which is the natural ability of the brain to learn how to accept movement without causing feelings of dizziness. However Dr. Timothy Hain debunks this idea in his 2017 post "Benzodiazepines in Dizziness—What is the Data?" where he reveals the studies that show these findings use extremely high doses that should never be prescribed for vestibular migraine. Your physician may prescribe the lowest dose before a flight. I personally recommend testing the dosage a few times in the comfort of your home so you can contact your physician if you need assistance, rather than testing medications on the day of your trip. If these are not an option for you, you can ask your doctor about over-the-counter medications like Dramamine or even Benadryl, which are also sometimes helpful.

Below are some additional tips to ease your journey while traveling with migraine:

- Do not to pack your medications in a checked suitcase. Keep them in your carry-on bag so you can be sure they are always with you.
- Choose a seat toward the front or over the wing of the plane. You'll feel less turbulence, and any motion changes won't be as drastic as they are in the back.
- If you do not think you can walk without assistance, arrange transportation from security to your gate. If notified of your illness, airlines will allow you to board early and get yourself situated with ease. Alerting the airline to your needs before your trip can help reduce a lot of fear. Planning ahead will calm anxiety.
- Find a scent you really enjoy that soothes you and bring along a small vial. I like peppermint or lavender essential oils. A dab under my nose and on my temples provides a nice cooling sensation and masks any unwanted smells. I've used this trick when someone next to me is wearing strong cologne or smells of smoke, and it works quite well.

- Plan for at least a day of adjusting time in a new city. This means no tours or big excursions—just some time to catch your breath. Traveling is a lot to handle for our sensitive brains, so having a day or two off is essential.

- FL-41 or tinted lenses can be incredibly helpful when navigating airports. Florescent lights and large windows, along with crowds of people and loud noises, can mean sensory overload. These lenses will help filter some of that light without being too dark and potentially increasing your light sensitivity, like sunglasses would.

- Beware of airplane food! Prepare ahead of time with snacks like the Pepita Protein Bars (page 116) or Seed Butter Energy Balls (page 131), plain potato or tortilla chips, apples, seeds, and cut vegetables. TSA will allow you to bring a cooler onboard, as long as the ice pack is frozen when you go through security. On long flights, I'll bring the pasta salad with me because it does well at room temperature.

- Hydrate—with water, not mini bottles of vodka. I bring an empty insulated bottle with me and fill it up once I'm through security. I love that it keeps my water cold, which makes me more inclined to keep drinking it.

- If anxiety is a huge issue for you, consider downloading meditations from the Calm app or playing hemi-sync music. Breathing techniques can also help keep that nervous energy from triggering more symptoms.

- Remember that traveling increases the number of triggers in your proverbial bucket. Keeping food and other triggers low will help you stay below that migraine attack threshold.

Support

Living with chronic migraine or a vestibular disorder can feel incredibly isolating. Even the kindest spouses and family members will never truly understand what you're experiencing. It's important to form a connection with someone who knows what you're going through. I highly recommend finding a support group to be a part of. There are a few online and in-person support groups through VeDA (Vestibular Disorders Association) and Miles for Migraine, as well as Facebook groups for migraine disorders, like Migraine Strong. My advice is to join a few groups, find the ones you really like where you feel supported, then leave or mute the others.

Many times, some of these groups can bring you down or begin to feel depressing. You must remember that the members in remission have probably all left these groups and are out living their lives! I've been told by multiple neurologists that remission is possible, and now I'm even getting a taste of it.

Find someone you connect with inside the group and see if they're open to messaging. A lot of my vestibular migraine buddies were people in my support groups, and they've become some of my closest friends. A few I have finally met in person!

For help with recipes, you can join The Dizzy Cook Recipe Chat on Facebook. Here you will find support or be able to ask questions about anything discussed in this book.

If you ever feel like this illness is too much to handle, please tell someone. Talk to a therapist, a friend, or your physician. Do not hesitate to call the National Suicide Prevention Lifeline should you ever need it: 1-800-273-8255.

For more delicious recipes and helpful tips, visit TheDizzyCook.com.

Research & Resources

"About Magtein." *Magtein.* AIDP. Accessed October 4, 2019. http://magtein.com/about.html

Alghadir, Ahmad H and Shahnawaz Anwer. "Effects of Vestibular Rehabilitation in the Management of a Vestibular Migraine: A Review." *Frontiers in neurology,* Vol 9 440. 2018. DOI:10.3389/fneur.2018.00440.

Beh, Shin C., et al. "The Spectrum of Vestibular Migraine: Clinical Features, Triggers, and Examination Findings." *Headache,* Vol 59. 2019. DOI: 10.1111/head.13484.

Beh, Shin C. and Deborah I. Friedman. "Vestibular Migraine." *University of Texas Southwestern Medical Center.* Dallas, Texas. https://americanheadachesociety.org/wp-content/uploads/2018/06/Beh-Vestibular-Migraine.docx

Buchholz, David. *Heal Your Headache: The 1-2-3 Program For Taking Charge of Your Pain.* Workman: New York, 2002.

Cha, Yoon-Hee. "Migraine-associated vertigo: diagnosis and treatment." *Seminars in neurology,* Vol 30, No 2: 167–174. 2010. DOI:10.1055/s-0030-1249225.

Cherchi, Marcello and Timothy C. Hain. "Nutritional supplements for Migraine." *Chicago Dizziness and Hearing.* September 1, 2019. https://www.dizziness-and-balance.com/disorders/central/migraine/treatments/migraine%20nutritional%20supplements.htm

Condo, Maria, et al. "Riboflavin prophylaxis in pediatric and adolescent migraine." *The Journal of Headache and Pain,* Vol 10, No 4: 361-5. 2009. DOI: 10.1007/s10194-009-0142-2.

Dimitrova, AK, RC Ungaro, B Lebwohl, et al. "Prevalence of migraine in patients with celiac disease and inflammatory bowel disease." *Headache,* Vol 53, No 2:344-55. February 2013. DOI: 10.1111/j.1526-4610.2012.02260.x.

Gröber, Uwe et al. "Myth or Reality-Transdermal Magnesium?." *Nutrients,* Vol. 9, No 8: 813. July 28, 2017, DOI:10.3390/nu9080813

Hain, Timothy C. "Benzodiazepines in dizziness - what is the data?" *Chicago Dizziness and Hearing.* November 18, 2017. https://www.dizziness-and-balance.com/treatment/drug/benzodiazepines%20in%20vertigo.html

Hain, Timothy C. "Vestibular Rehabilitation Therapy (VRT): For patients who have been referred for vestibular therapy." *Chicago Dizziness and Hearing.* September 18, 2017. https://dizziness-and-balance.com/treatment/rehab.html

Lempert, Thomas, et al. "Vestibular migraine: diagnostic criteria." *Journal of Vestibular Research* 2012, Vol 22, No 4: 167–172. DOI: 10.3233/VES-2012-0453.

Lin, Yu-Kai, et al. "Associations Between Sleep Quality and Migraine Frequency: A Cross-Sectional Case-Control Study." *Medicine* 2016, Vol 95, No 17. DOI: 10.1097/MD.0000000000003554.

Lindberg, JS, et al. "Magnesium bioavailability from magnesium citrate and magnesium oxide." *Journal of the American College of Nutrition,* Vol 9, No 1: 48-55. February 1990. DOI: 10.1080/07315724.1990.10720349.

Liu, Yuan F and Helen Xu. "The Intimate Relationship between Vestibular Migraine and Meniere Disease: A Review of Pathogenesis and Presentation." *Behavioural Neurology* 2016, Vol 2016, Article ID 3182735. DOI: 10.1155/2016/3182735.

"Low-Tyramine Diet for Migraine." *National Headache Foundation Blog.* 2019. https://headaches.org/2007/10/25/low-tyramine-diet-for-migraine/.

Maghbooli, Mehdi, et al. "Comparison Between the Efficacy of Ginger and Sumatriptan in the Ablative Treatment of the Common Migraine." *Phytotherapy Research* 2014, Vol 28, No 3: 412-5. DOI: 10.1002/ptr.4996.

Martin, VT and B Vij. "Diet and Headache: Part 1." *Headache,* Vol 56, No 9:1543-52. October 2016. DOI: 10.1111/head.12953.

Martins, Lais Bhering, et al. "Double-blind placebo-controlled randomized clinical trial of ginger (Zingiber officinale Rosc.) addition in migraine acute treatment." *Cephalalgia* 2019, Vol 39, No 1: 68-76. DOI: 10.1177/0333102418776016.

Mauskop, Alexander and Jasmine Varughese. "Why all migraine patients should be treated with magnesium." *Journal of Neural Transmission,* Vol 119, No 5: 575-9. May 2012. DOI: 10.1007/s00702-012-0790-2.

McCarty, MF. "Magnesium taurate and fish oil for prevention of migraine." *Medical Hypotheses,* Vol 47, No 6: 461-6. December 1996. DOI: 10.1016/s0306-9877(96)90158-9.

Neuhauser H, et al. "The interrelations of migraine, vertigo, and migrainous vertigo." *Neurology* 2001, Vol 56, No 4: 436-441. DOI: 10.1212/WNL.56.4.436.

Rozen, TD, et al. "Open label trial of coenzyme Q10 as a migraine preventative." *Cephalalgia* 2002, Vol 22, No 2: 137-41. DOI: 10.1046/j.1468-2982.2002.00335.x.

Schuette, Sally A, et al. "Bioavailability of magnesium diglycinate vs magnesium oxide in patients with ileal resection." *Journal of Parenteral and Enteral Nutrition* 1994, Vol 18, No 5: 430-5. DOI: 10.1177/0148607194018005430.

Teixido, Michael and John Carey. "Migraine: More Than a Headache." Johns Hopkins Otolaryngology-Head & Neck Surgery. May 14, 2014. https://www.hopkinsmedicine.org/otolaryngology/_docs/Migraine%20patient%20handout.pdf

Uysal, Nazan, et al. "Timeline (Bioavailability) of Magnesium Compounds in Hours: Which Magnesium Compound Works Best?" *Biological Trace Element Research,* Vol 187, No 1: 128-36. January 2019. DOI: 10.1007/s12011-018-1351-9.

Varkey, Emma, et al. "Exercise as migraine prophylaxis: a randomized study using relaxation and topiramate as controls." *Cephalalgia* 2001, Vol 13, No 14. DOI: 10.1177/0333102411419681.

Index

Note: Page references in *italics* indicate photographs.

Acknowledgments

To all of my TheDizzyCook.com readers, emailers, commenters, and recipe makers: thank you so much for inspiring me and encouraging me to be a better cook, writer, and researcher. Every comment or email I receive where someone says they cut their migraine days in half (or more!) because of my recipes and tips warms my heart. It pushes me to keep going, even when some days are extra hard.

To my husband, Casey, who is the best thing that ever happened to me. Thank you for all the late-night grocery runs, the countless dishes you washed, and for picking me up off the kitchen floor and giving me the greatest bear hugs every time I moaned that I couldn't possibly cook anymore. But most of all, thank you for believing that I was capable of something greater when I was stuck in my dead-end job and when I stayed on the couch for weeks at a time, too ill with this "mysterious illness" to even walk or drive. Every day I'm grateful that the way to your heart was, in fact, through your stomach. Also, sorry for all the times I yelled at you to get out of the fridge because all the food in it needed to be photographed.

To my family and friends, for all your support for this book, but also the countless doctors' appointments and making an effort to understand that vestibular migraine isn't just a headache. Mom & Dad, thank you for being proud of me even when I wasn't proud of myself. And Ann & Van, thank you for allowing me to take over the Wolf family Thanksgiving so I could test my recipes. Your excitement over this book means everything to me.

To my editor, Jen, whom I'm convinced is Superwoman and inspires me to be the best boss lady I can be, even with VM. You believed in me from the very beginning, and I could not be more honored that you chose to work with me. Thank you for your (very) gentle guidance, your encouragement, and your friendship. Rachel, Olivia, and Angie: thank you for also helping me bring this vision to life, and for doing it in such a beautiful way.

To all my migraine buddies, especially Jennifer and Kayla: I value the friendship we have built through an incredible hardship. If there's one positive thing that's come from this, it's knowing you guys and being able to lean on each other through the hard days. You both have helped me in so many ways with *The Dizzy Cook*, and I cannot thank you enough. Kayla McCain, you are a marketing genius and I owe you many meals as payment for all your help! Also the rest of my Migraine Strong team—Eileen, Danielle, and Marina—who have supported me since day one and taught me so much… and not just about migraine!

My deepest gratitude to Dr. Shin Beh and his team at UTSW for being the first doctor who didn't make me feel totally crazy. It's because of you I have "100% days" again. Thank you also to the other doctors who have furthered my education into this illness and become advocates for the VM community: Dr. Edward Cho, Dr. Timothy Hain, and Dr. Michael Teixido.

Dr. David Buchholz, your book gave me hope that I might live a normal life again. Thanks also to Paula, Carl, and the Migraine Again and MWS team for continuing to push for more education, awareness, and research into Migraine Disease. Last but definitely not least, VeDA. I have so much love for y'all and how you spread much-needed awareness about vestibular disorders, like Vestibular Migraine. I'm looking forward to the day that the IHS classifies Vestibular Migraine as an actual type of Migraine!

Thanks to Megan Weaver for making me look good, and to Erin Tindol for the beautiful photographs of Jennifer Bragdon, The Dizzy Baker.